FACILITATOR GUIDE

HIGH RELIABILITY ORGANIZATIONS
THIRD EDITION

A Healthcare Handbook for Patient Safety & Quality

CYNTHIA A. OSTER, PhD, MBA, APRN, ACNS-BC, CNS-BC, ANP, FAAN
JANE S. BRAATEN, PhD, APRN, CNS, ANP, CPPS, CPHQ

Contributors:
Noreen Bernard, EdD, RN, NEA-BC, FAAN
Kristen A. Oster, DNP, EMBA, APRN, ACNS-BC, CNOR, CNS-CP

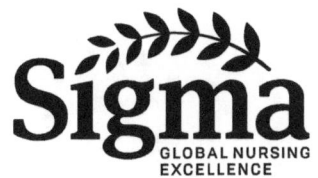

Copyright © 2026 by Sigma Theta Tau International Honor Society of Nursing

All rights reserved. This book is protected by copyright. No part of it may be reproduced, stored in a retrieval system, or transmitted in any form or by any means, electronic, mechanical, photocopying, recording, or otherwise, without written permission from the publisher. Any trademarks, service marks, design rights, or similar rights that are mentioned, used, or cited in this book are the property of their respective owners. Their use here does not imply that you may use them for a similar or any other purpose.

This book is not intended to be a substitute for the medical advice of a licensed medical professional. The author and publisher have made every effort to ensure the accuracy of the information contained within at the time of its publication and shall have no liability or responsibility to any person or entity regarding any loss or damage incurred, or alleged to have incurred, directly or indirectly, by the information contained in this book. The author and publisher make no warranties, express or implied, with respect to its content, and no warranties may be created or extended by sales representatives or written sales materials. The author and publisher have no responsibility for the consistency or accuracy of URLs and content of third-party websites referenced in this book.

Sigma Theta Tau International Honor Society of Nursing (Sigma) is a nonprofit organization whose mission is advancing world health and celebrating nursing excellence in scholarship, leadership, and service. Founded in 1922, Sigma has more than 90,000 active members in over 100 countries and territories. Members include practicing nurses, instructors, researchers, policymakers, entrepreneurs, and others. Sigma's more than 540 chapters are located at more than 700 institutions of higher education throughout Armenia, Australia, Botswana, Brazil, Canada, Colombia, England, Eswatini, Ghana, Hong Kong, Ireland, Israel, Jamaica, Japan, Jordan, Kenya, Lebanon, Malawi, Mexico, the Netherlands, Nigeria, Pakistan, Philippines, Portugal, Puerto Rico, Scotland, Singapore, South Africa, South Korea, Sweden, Taiwan, Tanzania, Thailand, the United States, and Wales. Learn more at www.sigmanursing.org.

Sigma Theta Tau International
550 West North Street
Indianapolis, IN, USA 46202

To request a review copy for course adoption, order additional books, buy in bulk, or purchase for corporate use, contact Sigma Marketplace at 888.654.4968 (US/Canada toll-free), +1.317.687.2256 (International), or solutions@sigmamarketplace.org.

To request author information, or for speaker or other media requests, contact Sigma Marketing at 888.634.7575 (US/Canada toll-free) or +1.317.634.8171 (International).

ISBN: 9781646481774
ISBN EPUB: 9781646481767
ISBN PDF: 9781646481644

Publisher: Dustin Sullivan
Acquisitions Editor: Emily Hatch
Development Editor: Jillmarie Leeper Sycamore
Cover Designer: Michael Tanamachi
Interior Design/Page Layout: Rebecca Batchelor

Managing Editor: Carla Hall
Project Editor: Todd Lothery
Copy Editor: Todd Lothery
Proofreader: Todd Lothery

ACKNOWLEDGMENTS

The authors wish to thank Noreen Bernard and Kristen Oster for contributing their expertise and clinical experiences to make this guide relevant to both instructor and student.

ABOUT THE EDITORS

Cynthia A. Oster, PhD, MBA, APRN, ACNS-BC, CNS-BC, ANP, FAAN, is the Enterprise Nurse Scientist—Research Program Manager for the Mountain Region of CommonSpirit Health in Centennial, Colorado, following four years of service as the Patient Safety Nurse Scientist at Emory Healthcare and adjunct Assistant Professor at the Nell Hodgson Woodruff School of Nursing at Emory University in Atlanta, Georgia. For more than a decade, Oster was a nurse scientist for Centura Health and a clinical nurse specialist for critical care and cardiovascular services at AdventHealth Porter in Denver, Colorado. She has held research, clinical, educational, and administrative positions throughout her more than 40-year career. Oster received her BSN from the University of Iowa, her MSN from the University of Nebraska Medical Center, and her PhD from the University of Colorado College of Nursing. In addition, she earned an ANP certificate from Beth El College of Nursing in Colorado Springs, Colorado, and an MBA from the University of Colorado-Denver. She holds Clinical Nurse Specialist-Core and Adult Clinical Nurse Specialist certification from the American Nurses Credentialing Center. In 2017, she became a Fellow in the American Academy of Nursing. She mentors clinical nurses and advanced practice nurses to develop clinical practice wisdom through application of high reliability principles, evidence-based practice, and the conduct of research. Oster has presented at national and international meetings and has published in the areas of high reliability, evidence-based practice, alarm fatigue, and peer review. She is a member of Sigma Theta Tau International, the American Nurses Association, the American Association of Critical-Care Nurses, the National Association of Clinical Nurse Specialists, the American College of Healthcare Executives, and Beta Gamma Sigma.

Jane S. Braaten, PhD, APRN, CNS, ANP, CPPS, CPHQ, is a Regional Director of Patient Safety and High Reliability at CommonSpirit Health in Centennial, Colorado. She has held positions as Director of Cardiology Services, Cardiac and Intensive Care Clinical Nurse Specialist, Cardiac Nurse Practitioner, and Manager/Charge RN/Staff RN of intensive care and telemetry units. Braaten obtained her BSN from the Indiana University School of Nursing and holds the degree of doctor of philosophy, a master's degree as a clinical nurse specialist, and a certificate as an adult nurse practitioner from the University of Colorado College of Nursing. She also is a certified professional in patient safety (CPPS) and a certified professional in healthcare quality (CPHQ). She has presented at national meetings and has published in the areas of hospital system barriers to rapid response team activation, quality improvement in telemetry, end-of-life care in the intensive care unit, leadership, and high reliability organizations and healthcare. She is a passionate mentor and supporter to those at the front line who create safe patient care daily.

ABOUT THE CONTRIBUTORS

Noreen Bernard, EdD, RN, NEA-BC, FAAN, is a distinguished nurse executive with extensive experience in shaping nursing practice across both acute care and ambulatory settings. As a Chief Nursing Officer overseeing multiple sites within a prominent health system, Bernard excels in executive systems leadership, clinical operations, and workforce strategies, driving nursing excellence and enhancing professional practice. Her commitment to high reliability is reflected in her focus on improving quality and patient safety outcomes. In addition to her executive role, Bernard contributes to academia as an adjunct faculty member and doctoral program content expert at two universities. Her scholarly work spans several critical areas, including nursing administration, resilience, job satisfaction, professional joy, leader development, and nursing practice. Bernard is also actively involved in the academic community as a volunteer editor and board member for three national journals. Bernard earned her doctor of education in organizational leadership and organization development from Grand Canyon University, her master's in nursing administration from the University of Colorado, and her BSN from the University of Northern Colorado. She is Nurse Executive Advanced Board Certified and was honored as a Fellow in the American Academy of Nursing in 2019. Her professional journey reflects a steadfast dedication to advancing the field of nursing through leadership, research, and education.

Kristen A. Oster, DNP, EMBA, APRN, ACNS-BC, CNOR, CNS-CP, is currently the Director of Surgical Services at Intermountain Health Good Samaritan Hospital in Lafayette, Colorado. She has held a variety of perioperative and ambulatory positions throughout her career, including operating room and pain procedural care clinical manager; assistant nurse manager for an ENT, skull base, head/neck, and neurosurgery service line; perioperative clinical nurse specialist; clinical manager for geographic float pools; and regional nursing services coordinator supporting ambulatory services. She was the Patient Safety Specialist assigned to the perioperative and ambulatory service line at the University of Colorado–Anschutz Medical Campus in Aurora, Colorado. She received a bachelor of science degree in biology and education from Denison University in Granville, Ohio. Oster earned a bachelor of science degree in nursing from the accelerated nursing program at Regis University, Denver, Colorado. She holds a master of science in nursing degree—clinical nurse specialist focus in adult and geriatric acute care and Doctorate in Nursing Practice—from the University of Colorado, Denver. She completed her executive master's in business administration at the University of Colorado, Denver. Oster is a member of the Association of periOperative Registered Nurses and American Organization of Nursing Leadership.

TABLE OF CONTENTS

About the Editors iv
About the Contributors v
Introduction x

UNIT 1 USING THE TEXTBOOK FOR TEACHING AND LEARNING 2

    CONSISTENCY WITH NURSING EDUCATION ACCREDITATION STANDARDS 3

    STRATEGIES FOR TEACHING 5

UNIT 2 RESOURCES FOR TEACHING HIGH RELIABILITY FOR PATIENT SAFETY AND QUALITY 7

    EVIDENCE-BASED PRACTICE (EBP) RESOURCES 8

    CHANGE MANAGEMENT MODELS 8

    INFLUENTIAL RESOURCES ON HROs 8

    NATIONAL RESOURCES FOR QUALITY AND PATIENT SAFETY 9

UNIT 3 CHAPTER LEARNING ACTIVITIES AND FACILITATOR SUPPORT ... 11

    PART I HIGH RELIABILITY: THE IMPERATIVE REMAINS 12

        1 HIGH RELIABILITY: REFLECTIONS ON THE ESSENCE OF HRO AND THE APPLICATION TO HEALTHCARE 13

        Learning Activity 1.1: Compare and Contrast External/Internal Drivers Shaping the Healthcare Quality and Safety Paradigm Shift 14

        2 DRIVERS FOR PATIENT SAFETY 17

        Learning Activity 2.1: Differentiate Individual and System Factors Within Patient Harm Events Through Application of High Reliability Principles to Discover Solutions and Explore Barriers 18

        3 CURRENT QUALITY DRIVERS 20

        Learning Activity 3.1: Discover How Evidence-Based Practice Aligns With High Reliability Principles to Inform Drivers of Quality 21

        4 ORGANIZATIONAL CULTURE AND PSYCHOLOGICAL SAFETY: BREAKING DOWN BARRIERS 26

        Learning Activity 4.1: Compare and Contrast Facilitators and Barriers of Psychological Safety and Discuss Practical Measures of Psychological Safety 27

        5 SAFETY LEADERSHIP: COMMITMENT TO HIGH RELIABILITY ORGANIZING ... 30

        Learning Activity 5.1: Compare and Contrast Characteristics of Safety Leadership Styles and Safety Leadership Actions Within a High Reliability Organizing Framework 31

6   HEALTH EQUITY AND HIGH RELIABILITY: CONNECTING THE DOTS FOR PATIENT SAFETY..... 37

Learning Activity 6.1: Use Health Equity Knowledge to Inform Patient Safety Initiatives 38

PART II   HRO CONCEPTS AND APPLICATION TO PRACTICE: PREOCCUPATION WITH FAILURE 41

7   USING FAILURE MODE AND EFFECTS ANALYSIS TO PREDICT FAILURE 42

Learning Activity 7.1: Discuss the Importance of the FMEA Process Within a High Reliability Organization 43

8   PAYING ATTENTION TO CLOSE CALLS AND NEAR MISSES 46

Learning Activity 8.1: Evaluate the Importance of Near Misses, Close Calls, and Unsafe Conditions to High Reliability 47

PART III   HRO CONCEPTS AND APPLICATION TO PRACTICE: RELUCTANCE TO SIMPLIFY 49

9   HUMAN FACTORS ENGINEERING FOR REDUCING AND RECOVERING FROM ERROR 50

Learning Activity 9.1: Explain Human Factors Engineering (HFE): The Science and Practice of Designing Work Systems to Fit the Needs, Limitations, and Capabilities of Humans 51

10   ROOT CAUSE ANALYSIS: A TOOL FOR HIGH RELIABILITY IN A COMPLEX ENVIRONMENT 55

Learning Activity 10.1: Discuss Use of RCA as a Tool for Embedding the High Reliability Principle "Reluctance to Simplify" Into a Safety Event Investigation 56

11   FOSTERING JUST CULTURE IN HIGH RELIABILITY ORGANIZATIONS: HOW FAR HAVE WE COME? 59

Learning Activity 11.1: Examine the Features and Challenges of a Just Culture Within a Highly Reliable Safety Program and the Current Healthcare Environment 60

PART IV   HRO CONCEPTS AND APPLICATION TO PRACTICE: SENSITIVITY TO OPERATIONS 64

12   ALARM SAFETY: WORKING SOLUTIONS 65

Learning Activity 12.1: Appraise the Concept of Alarm Fatigue and the Possibilities for Improvement When Applying High Reliability Principles to Clinical Alarm Safety 66

13   INNOVATIVE TECHNOLOGY, STANDARDIZATION, AND THE IMPACT ON HIGH RELIABILITY 68

Learning Activity 13.1: Apply Knowledge of Effective Interventions for High Reliability to Analyze Technological Advances in Your Practice 69

14 TIERED SAFETY HUDDLES ... 73
Learning Activity 14.1: Describe the Value of the Tiered Huddle in Healthcare as an Effective Tool to Promote High Reliability in a Complex Organization ... 74

PART V HRO CONCEPTS AND APPLICATION TO PRACTICE: DEFERENCE TO EXPERTISE ... 76

15 THE CURRENT NEED FOR INTERPROFESSIONAL COLLABORATIVE CARE AND TEAMWORK ... 77
Learning Activity 15.1: Describe and Explain an Interprofessional Team in the Context of HROs ... 78

16 MEANINGFUL PATIENT ENGAGEMENT: BEST PRACTICE FOR HIGH RELIABILITY ... 81
Learning Activity 16.1: Explain Meaningful Patient and Family Engagement in the Context of High Reliability for Patient Safety and Quality ... 82

17 PEDIATRIC PATIENT SAFETY: UTILIZING SAFETY COACHING AS A STRATEGY TOWARD ZERO HARM ... 84
Learning Activity 17.1: Examine the Role of Safety Coaches as a Vehicle for Successful Change Management and Sustainability of HRO Principles ... 85

PART VI HRO CONCEPTS AND APPLICATION TO PRACTICE: COMMITMENT TO RESILIENCE ... 88

18 DESIGNING RESILIENCE INTO THE WORK ENVIRONMENT ... 89
Learning Activity 18.1: Apply a Social-Ecological Perspective of Resilience to Support Clinician Well-Being in the Work Environment ... 90

19 BUILDING HIGH RELIABILITY THROUGH SIMULATION ... 93
Learning Activity 19.1: Explore Opportunities to Use Simulation to Improve Safety and Reliability of Risk-Prone Processes ... 94

20 BUILDING RESILIENCE THROUGH TEAM TRAINING: RAPID RESPONSE AND IN-HOSPITAL CARDIAC ARREST EVENTS ... 96
Learning Activity 20.1: Evaluate Rapid Response and In-Hospital Cardiac Arrest Event Team Performance ... 97

21 SUSTAINING A CULTURE OF SAFETY ... 100
Learning Activity 21.1: Focus on Sustaining a Culture of Safety in a Resilient Organization ... 101

PART VII ASSIMILATION INTO PRACTICE ACROSS THE CONTINUUM ... 104

22 AMBULATORY CARE: THE FRONTIER FOR HIGH RELIABILITY ... 105
Learning Activity 22.1: Integrate High Reliability Principles to Address Quality and Safety Challenges in Ambulatory Care ... 106

23 THE SYNTHESIS AMONG MAGNET RECOGNITION PROGRAM® MODEL COMPONENTS AND HIGH RELIABILITY ORGANIZATION PRINCIPLES 108

Learning Activity 23.1: Explain the Synergistic Relationship Between the Magnet Model Components and the Principles of High Reliability 109

24 REALIZING HIGH RELIABILITY: NURSE SCIENTIST AND BEDSIDE SCIENTIST COLLABORATION 112

Learning Activity 24.1: Discover the Role of the Nurse Scientist and Bedside Scientist in a High Reliability Organization 113

25 ENSURING HIGH RELIABILITY IN ACUTE STROKE TREATMENT 119

Learning Activity 25.1: Apply High Reliability Principles to Acute Stroke Treatment 120

PART VIII TRANSLATION INTO PRACTICE 122

26 HIGH RELIABILITY PERFORMANCE DURING A PANDEMIC 123

Learning Activity 26.1: Explore High Reliability Performance During a Pandemic 124

27 BUILDING A HIGH RELIABILITY HEAD AND NECK OPERATING ROOM TEAM 126

Learning Activity 27.1: Apply High Reliability Principles to Solve Team Quality and Safety Challenges 127

28 DECREASING HARM FROM WORKPLACE VIOLENCE 131

Learning Activity 28.1: Discuss Causes, Consequences, and Interventions to Workplace Violence in Healthcare 132

29 INTRODUCTION OF HIGH RELIABILITY TO FRONTLINE STAFF: CREATING A VIRTUAL RESOURCE TOOLKIT 134

Learning Activity 29.1: Apply High Reliability Principles to Solve Organizational Team Quality and Safety Challenges 135

PART IX TRANSLATION INTO PRACTICE SUMMATIVE ASSESSMENT 139

SUMMATIVE ASSESSMENT: TRANSLATION INTO PRACTICE 140

Summative Assessment Learning Activity: Translate Evidence-Based Practice, Change Management, and High Reliability Principles to Practice 141

SUPPLEMENTAL FACILITATOR RESOURCES AND READINGS 144

APPENDICES 152

A EBP WORKSHEET 153

B HIGH RELIABILITY ORGANIZATIONS: A QUICK GUIDE FOR FRONTLINE APPLICATION 156

What Are High Reliability Organizations (HROs)? 157
High Reliability Organization Characteristics* 158

INTRODUCTION

Welcome to the *Facilitator Guide for High Reliability Organizations: A Healthcare Handbook for Patient Safety & Quality*, 3rd Edition. This guide is designed to be a resource for educators in a variety of academic settings in courses focused on patient safety or quality management in nursing, health services administration, or clinical programs.

ABOUT THE FACILITATOR GUIDE

This facilitator guide is divided into three sections:

- **Unit 1:** Using the Textbook for Teaching and Learning
- **Unit 2:** Resources for Teaching High Reliability for Patient Safety and Quality
- **Unit 3:** Chapter Learning Activities and Facilitator Support

This guide provides suggestions to guide faculty, nurse leaders, clinical staff nurses, quality and safety staff, or other healthcare professionals who are teaching others about the application of HRO principles to patient safety and quality problems using the 3rd edition of *High Reliability Organizations: A Healthcare Handbook for Patient Safety & Quality*. For academic faculty, the chapter-by-chapter learning activities will help facilitate student learning about application of high reliability to patient safety and quality and can be used as part of a patient safety and quality course at a variety of academic levels.

The companion *Workbook for High Reliability Organizations: A Healthcare Handbook for Patient Safety & Quality* (3rd ed.) contains the same chapter-by-chapter learning activities found in this facilitator guide. The facilitator guide contains supplemental materials including learning activity implementation strategies and student evaluation sections. There are several completed examples of fill-in responses or answers for facilitators as well. A summative learning activity is included that gives facilitators the opportunity to assess student ability to translate high reliability principles into practice.

ABOUT THE BOOK

High Reliability Organizations comprehensively describes how to infuse the knowledge, skills, and attitudes of an HRO into the fabric of an organization from the boardroom to the front lines of care, including patients and their families. The book is based on the premise that although a quest for high reliability must start in the boardroom, it must also be part of every person's focus. The current message in patient safety and quality literature is that we, in healthcare, need to strive to be highly reliable, meaning that we should be a system that detects and prevents errors from happening even though we operate in high-risk, emergent conditions. Most often, the conversation goes in the direction that healthcare should be similar to aviation. This message is not helpful to healthcare providers as they strive to understand what high reliability is and looks like in the healthcare field.

The textbook addresses that gap by providing an understanding of HRO and the application of its concepts to clinical practice. Practical examples are offered that support each of the five concepts of HRO along with useful tools, measurements, and design strategies. The various chapters tease apart the multiple facets of HROs and apply the standards to everyday components of care. Chapter content blends leadership approaches with frontline clinician application. The text places the need for high reliability concepts into our current climate in healthcare through illustrative discussion (theory and research) of each of the five concepts of HRO, along with a description of a current best practice or tool that applies to the model. As a tool for teaching and learning the course textbook, it explains in Part I how high reliability provides the background for the current safety and quality environment. It recommends in Parts II through VI HRO concepts as a framework for quality and safety activities. In Parts VII and VIII, it integrates high reliability principles into healthcare practice across the care continuum. Part IX provides a summative course assessment. Although we do not intend this as a textbook, it could be used in graduate courses focused on patient safety or quality management in nursing, health services administration, or clinical programs.

UNIT 1
USING THE TEXTBOOK FOR TEACHING AND LEARNING

CONSISTENCY WITH NURSING EDUCATION ACCREDITATION STANDARDS

Nursing faculty may use the textbook, the facilitator guide, and the workbook to facilitate meeting of accreditation standards related to quality care and patient safety in the curriculum. The major accreditation standards relating to quality care and patient safety content are:

- American Association of Colleges of Nursing
- National League for Nursing
- Accreditation Commission for Education in Nursing

American Association of Colleges of Nursing

The American Association of Colleges of Nursing (AACN) is the driving force for innovation and excellence in academic nursing and publishes the *Essentials* series. The *Essentials* series delineates the national consensus by providing the elements and framework for building nursing curricula. The Essentials outline the necessary curriculum content and expected competencies of graduates from baccalaureate, master's, and DNP programs, as well as the clinical support needed for the full spectrum of academic nursing. These are public domain documents and are easily retrievable. Mentions of quality and patient safety are found explicitly in the following:

- *The Essentials of Baccalaureate Education for Professional Nursing Practice* (2008). Essential II: Basic Organizational and Systems Leadership for Quality Care and Patient Safety recognizes that a baccalaureate-prepared nurse must possess the knowledge and skills in leadership, quality improvement, and patient safety that are necessary to provide high-quality healthcare, including reliability and reliability sciences in healthcare. http://www.aacnnursing.org/portals/42/publications/baccessentials08.pdf

- *The Essentials of Master's Education in Nursing* (2011). Essential III: Quality Improvement and Safety recognizes that a master's-prepared nurse must be articulate in the methods, tools, performance measures, and standards related to quality and safety, as well as prepared to apply quality and safety principles within an organization, including using high reliability principles. http://www.aacnnursing.org/portals/42/publications/mastersessentials11.pdf

- *The Essentials of Doctoral Education for Advanced Nursing Practice* (2006). Essential II: Organizational and Systems Leadership for Quality Improvement and Systems Thinking recognizes that organizational and systems leadership are critical for DNP graduates to improve patient and healthcare outcomes. Doctoral-level knowledge and skills in these areas ensure accountability for quality of healthcare and patient safety for populations with whom they work. Essential III: Clinical Scholarship and Analytical Methods for Evidence-Based Practice recognizes that DNP graduates engage in advanced nursing practice and provide leadership for evidence-based practice (EBP). This requires competence in knowledge application activities: the translation of research in practice, the evaluation of practice, improvement of the reliability of healthcare practice, and outcomes and participation in collaborative research. https://www.aacnnursing.org/Portals/42/Publications/DNPEssentials.pdf

National League for Nursing

The National League for Nursing (NLN) promotes excellence in nursing education to build a strong and diverse nursing workforce that contributes to healthcare quality and safety and advances the health of our nation and the global community. The NLN Commission for Nursing Education Accreditation (CNEA) demonstrates that programs meet rigorous standards that foster continuous quality improvement in nursing programs and promote excellence in nursing education. The NLN CNEA promotes excellence and integrity in nursing education globally through an accreditation process that respects the diversity of program mission, curricula, students, and faculty; emphasizes a culture of continuous quality improvement; and influences the preparation of a caring and skilled nursing workforce.

Mentions of quality and patient safety are found explicitly in *CNEA Accreditation Standards for Nursing Education Programs* (2021). Mention of high reliability is not obvious; however, general reference of quality and safety is found in "Standard V: Culture of Learning and Diversity—Curriculum and Evaluation Processes." A curriculum integrating "context and environment of care delivery, knowledge and science applied to implementation and evaluation of evidenced-base care, personal and professional development, quality and safety, patient-centered care, and teamwork" is related to high reliability. https://irp.cdn-website.com/cc12ee87/files/uploaded/CNEA%20Standards%20October%202021-4b271cb2.pdf

Accreditation Commission for Education in Nursing

The Accreditation Commission for Education in Nursing (ACEN) supports the interests of nursing education, nursing practice, and the public by providing specialized accreditation for all levels of nursing education and transition-to-practice programs. The goal of the ACEN is to be a supportive partner in strengthening the quality of nursing education and transition-to-practice programs, and the commission is recognized as an accrediting body by the US Department of Education (USDE) and by the Council for Higher Education Accreditation (CHEA). ACEN accredits all types of nursing education programs—practical, diploma, associate, baccalaureate, master's including master's certificate, and clinical doctorate including DNP specialist certificate programs. ACEN accredits transition-to-practice programs that promote excellence in nursing and patient outcomes through established policies, procedures, and processes that are transparent, guided by peers and contemporary practice, and have an intentional focus on outcomes.

Mentions of quality and patient safety are implied in the following:

- ACEN Nursing Education 2023 Standards and Criteria. This document contains no overt reference of student learning outcomes specific to high reliability, quality, and patient safety. However, curriculum standard 4. 9 reflects this: "clinical/practicum learning environments and experiences reflect evidence-based nursing practice." https://resources.acenursing.org/space/SAC/1824227333/2023+Standards+and+Criteria?attachment=%2Fdownload%2Fattachments%2F1824227333%2F2023-Standards-and-Criteria-02282024.pdf&type=application%2Fpdf&filename=2023-Standards-and-Criteria-02282024.pdf

- ACEN Transition-To-Practice 2024 Standards and Criteria. There are no overt outcomes specific to high reliability, quality, and patient safety. However, curriculum standard 4.3 reflects this: "The curriculum enables the nurse resident to develop professional identity and independently assume the responsibilities of stated roles in leadership, professionalism, and safe clinical practice." https://resources.acenursing.org/space/Transition/1977974789/TTP+Standards+and+Criteria

STRATEGIES FOR TEACHING

There are several textbooks and scholarly articles on teaching strategies to facilitate the instruction and education of students. The following discussion is intended to supplement, not replace, these resources.

TEACHING STRATEGIES USEFUL IN TEACHING A HIGH RELIABILITY COURSE

Integration of real-world scenarios and student experiences into learning activities is a unique and useful teaching strategy for high reliability. Experiential learning translates high reliability concepts into reality, thus preparing the student to meet the national curriculum standards mentioned previously. Healthcare providers strive to understand what high reliability is and what it looks like in the healthcare field. Leveraging real practice situations provides accurate context for students to apply high reliability curriculum content and be able to see how high reliability can make a measurable difference in the practice environment.

STRATEGY IN THE CLASSROOM

In the physical classroom, engagement is essential. The flipped classroom (FC) supports improvement of critical thinking and problem-solving skills in students. In the FC, students learn foundational information outside of the classroom via reading assignments or watching prerecorded facilitator videos. In the classroom, students engage in activities that enhance foundational information via role play, case scenarios, games, simulation, and group discussion. The goal of flipped learning is for the facilitator to clarify, improve, and supplement the knowledge learned independently by students outside of the classroom and enhance problem-solving and critical thinking skills. The use of discussion boards can be useful. Discussion boards can be a beneficial platform to field questions and post announcements between classes.

STRATEGY FOR DISTANCE (ONLINE) CLASSES

The engagement of students in an online class is essential, whether the class is synchronous or asynchronous. The goal of either is to ensure students are engaged with the learning process so they perceive they are part of the learning process and, as a result, retain the material and feel engaged in the distance learning environment.

Synchronous online learning offers students instantaneous feedback, the opportunity to see their classmates, and the ability to feel more engaged in the online experience. Students are able to ask questions based on content being discussed in the classroom and can raise questions based on their own experiences or readings. Opportunities for engagement may include the following:

- Brainstorming
- Role-playing/practice
- Partner paired exercises with a large group debrief
- Small group exercises with a large group debrief
- Use of the "what, so what, now what" learning protocol

- Appreciative inquiry
- Reflective learning with small or large group debrief
- Case study presentation
- Teach-back (peer-to-peer teaching/learning)

The advantage of synchronous learning is that students feel like talking and engage more with their peers. In addition to improved social interaction with peers, students can monitor classmates' reactions during discussions that can motivate students to continue engaging with their peers. Students appreciate receiving instantaneous feedback, are able to observe visual cues from peers, and feel a social connection in their online courses. Students feel a decrease in transactional distance. Thus, students do not necessarily need to be in the physical presence of other students to learn and feel a sense of accomplishment.

Asynchronous online learning allows students to take time to consider their thoughts, engage with the content more deeply, feel a part of the learning community, and post more reflective comments in discussion boards. Asynchronous interaction allows students to interact on their own schedule. Opportunities for engagement may include the following:

- Discussion boards for students to ask the following:
    - General questions about material/content
    - Questions about specific assignments
- Blogs or other types of posts
- Graded discussion boards as a response to a facilitator-guided question
- Other kinds of technology that are supported by the online platform, such as a PowerPoint presentation, paper, or group project submission that requires peer feedback, either written or verbal/recorded

The advantage of asynchronous learning dialogue is the flexibility it provides for anytime-anywhere e-learning, which is the main convenience of online learning. Students are able to contemplate the content before responding in discussion boards, thereby increasing cognitive engagement with the content, especially if the content is perceived as difficult. Asynchronous online learning enables students time to reflect on their own ideas as well as their peers to interact more deeply with the content.

UNIT 2

RESOURCES FOR TEACHING HIGH RELIABILITY FOR PATIENT SAFETY AND QUALITY

A variety of resources are available that can assist the facilitator and enrich the student experience. Applying HRO principles to clinical problems and understanding how evidence-based practice and change management methods are integrated within the umbrella of quality and safety improvement are essential. The following is a list and description of resources.

EVIDENCE-BASED PRACTICE (EBP) RESOURCES

The student and facilitator need to be familiar with EBP. The student will need to be able to choose a model and apply it to a practice problem within the context of HRO. Resources include:

- Cullen, L., Hanrahan, K., Farrington, M., Tucker, S., & Edmonds, S. (2022). *Evidence-based practice in action: Comprehensive strategies, tools, and tips from the University of Iowa Hospitals and Clinics*. Sigma Theta Tau International.

- Johns Hopkins model. https://www.hopkinsmedicine.org/evidence-based-practice/model-tools

- JBI EBP resources. A comprehensive toolkit for implementation of EBP. https://jbi.global/

- *Journal of Nursing Care Quality*. Journal recognized for application and publication of quality improvement and EBP projects as well as research. Great source for practical application examples. https://journals.lww.com/jncqjournal/pages/default.aspx

CHANGE MANAGEMENT MODELS

The student and facilitator need to be familiar with change management. The student will need to choose a model and apply it to a practice problem within the context of HRO. Resources include:

- Batras, D., Duff, C., & Smith, B. (2014). Organizational change theory: Implications for health promotion practice. *Health Promotion International*, *31*(1), 231–241. https://academic.oup.com/heapro/article/31/1/231/2355918

- Kotter Change Management 8 Step model. https://www.kotterinc.com/methodology/8-steps/

- Small, A., Gist, D., Souza, D., Dalton, J., Magny-Normilus, C., & David, D. (2016). Using Kotter's change model for implementing bedside handoff: A quality improvement project. *Journal of Nursing Care Quality*, *31*(4), 304–309. https://www.nursingcenter.com/journalarticle?Article_ID=3639513

- Udod, S., & Wagner, J. (2018). Common change theories and application to different nursing situations. In J. Wagner (Ed.), *Leadership and influencing change in nursing*. https://pressbooks.pub/leadershipandinfluencingchangeinnursing/chapter/chapter-9-common-change-theories-and-application-to-different-nursing-situations/

INFLUENTIAL RESOURCES ON HROs

Facilitators will find that the seminal works of Karl Weick and Kathleen Sutcliffe provide a basis for understanding the philosophy and research that led to the HRO principles highlighted in this book. Resources include:

- Weick, K., & Sutcliffe, K. (2007). *Managing the unexpected: Resilient performance in an age of uncertainty* (2nd ed.). Jossey-Bass.

- Weick, K., & Sutcliffe, K. (2015). *Managing the unexpected: Sustained performance in a complex world* (3rd ed.). Jossey-Bass.

NATIONAL RESOURCES FOR QUALITY AND PATIENT SAFETY

The following sections highlight a number of national resources that are available to help understand quality and patient safety.

AHRQ

The Agency for Healthcare Research and Quality (AHRQ) is a federal agency whose mission is to improve the nation's healthcare system. The AHRQ website contains educational materials, research, data sources, and toolkits for improvement. The AHRQ also offers funding and grants for patient safety and quality research.

- https://www.ahrq.gov/
- https://www.ahrq.gov/patient-safety/resources/index.html
- https://www.ahrq.gov/teamstepps-program/index.html

ECRI and ISMP

ECRI is a nonprofit organization that focuses on safety and quality and the impact of technology. It recently acquired the Institute for Safe Medication Practices (ISMP), a national leader in proactive safety in all phases of the medication delivery process.

- https://www.ecri.org/
- https://www.ismp.org/newsletters

IHI

The Institute for Healthcare Improvement (IHI) website contains a plethora of resources for improving care. The site contains white papers, toolkits, education, and innovations, and it is the certifying body for the Certified Professional in Patient Safety (CPPS) credential.

- http://www.ihi.org/about/Pages/default.aspx
- http://www.ihi.org/Topics/PatientSafety/Pages/default.aspx
- http://www.ihi.org/resources/Pages/Tools/Patient-Safety-Essentials-Toolkit.aspx
- http://www.ihi.org/resources/Pages/Tools/RCA2-Improving-Root-Cause-Analyses-and-Actions-to-Prevent-Harm.aspx
- http://www.ihi.org/education/cpps-certified-professional-in-patient-safety/Pages/default.aspx

NAM

The National Academy of Medicine, formerly the Institute of Medicine, is an evidence-based, independent scientific advisor whose mission is to improve health for all by advancing science, accelerating health equity, and providing independent, authoritative, and trusted advice nationally and globally (https://nam.edu/).

NQF

The National Quality Forum (NQF) is a nonprofit organization that specializes in data measurement and endorses and develops quality metrics (http://www.qualityforum.org/Home.aspx).

QSEN

Quality and Safety Education for Nurses (QSEN) is an institute committed to excellence in teaching quality and patient safety for nursing. The website includes toolkits, teaching aides, and research (https://qsen.org/).

TJC

The Joint Commission (TJC) is an international driver of quality and patient safety. TJC provides healthcare systems accreditation, quality and safety assessment, and improvement innovations.

- https://www.jointcommission.org/
- https://www.jointcommission.org/standards/national-patient-safety-goals/

UNIT 3

CHAPTER LEARNING ACTIVITIES AND FACILITATOR SUPPORT

Unit 3 provides chapter-by-chapter learning activities aligned with the book chapters. The same learning activities are furnished in the workbook. In addition, Unit 3 provides facilitator support. Each learning activity is followed by "Learning Activity Implementation" guidance, which includes suggestions and instructions for facilitator use. The "Learning Activity Implementation" section is followed by a "Student Evaluation" section that provides recommendations for the facilitator to evaluate the student's performance on the learning activity.

PART I

HIGH RELIABILITY: THE IMPERATIVE REMAINS

Learning Objective

Explain how high reliability contributes to organizational quality and safety (*analyzing*).

Contents

Chapter 1	High Reliability: Reflections on the Essence of HRO and the Application to Healthcare	13
Chapter 2	Drivers for Patient Safety	17
Chapter 3	Current Quality Drivers	20
Chapter 4	Organizational Culture and Psychological Safety: Breaking Down Barriers	26
Chapter 5	Safety Leadership: Commitment to High Reliability Organizing	30
Chapter 6	Health Equity and High Reliability: Connecting the Dots for Patient Safety	37

CHAPTER 1

HIGH RELIABILITY: REFLECTIONS ON THE ESSENCE OF HRO AND THE APPLICATION TO HEALTHCARE

In this chapter, students will learn how high reliability has evolved over the years and the challenges still facing healthcare as we strive to create highly reliable environments. Students will also learn about internal and external challenges facing healthcare and the essence of high reliability.

Learning Objective

Discuss the depth of the message of high reliability and the contributors essential to creating a successful HRO environment.

Learning Activity 1.1: Compare and Contrast External/Internal Drivers Shaping the Healthcare Quality and Safety Paradigm Shift

Learning Activity Objectives

1.1 Compare external and internal drivers of quality and safety in the current healthcare system (*analyzing*).

1.2 Explain high reliability and barriers to successful HRO application (*understanding*).

1.3 Describe a current application of high reliability that has produced relevant safety outcomes (*applying*).

Preparation

Prior to completion of the learning activity, students should:

- Read Chapter 1.
- Read "High Reliability Organizing in Healthcare: Still a Long Way Left to Go" at https://doi.org/10.1136/bmjqs-2021-014141.

Instructions

1.1 Create a table for internal and external drivers in healthcare (see Table 1.1). Discuss how these drivers affect quality and patient safety at both the system and the unit level.

Answer Example:

TABLE 1.1 INTERNAL AND EXTERNAL DRIVERS IN HEALTHCARE

External Drivers	Definition	Example	Macro Impact on Healthcare System	Micro Impact on Healthcare Facility (unit)
Regulation	Efforts to meet regulatory requirements to affect how we approach quality	Joint Commission and CMS safety and quality requirements	Affects reimbursement, certification, and functioning of the hospital system	Requires constant oversight of changing rules

Internal Drivers	Definition	Example	Macro Impact on Healthcare System	Micro Impact on Healthcare Facility
Zero harm	The internal goal to prevent serious safety events	Zero hospital-acquired infections	Need standardized tools and resources to meet this goal	Requires constant oversight and visible data

1.2 Compare and contrast how application of high reliability varies in understanding. Discuss an "artifact" of high reliability in your organization and how it encourages high reliability thinking.

1.3 Present an article from the literature using at least one principle of high reliability in a healthcare setting. Include the following in the discussion: Identify the high reliability principle, define the high reliability principle, and explain how the high reliability principle was applied in the article.

LEARNING ACTIVITY IMPLEMENTATION

Students will benefit most from the learning activities by working individually rather than in a group.

For Exercise 1.1, facilitators should guide students to use the templates provided and direct students to be prepared to discuss how internal and external drivers affect quality and patient safety at both the system and the unit level.

For Exercise 1.2, students should be able to distinguish between various applications of high reliability. Students should identify an "artifact" of high reliability in their organization and be prepared to articulate how the "artifact" encourages high reliability thinking in the organization.

Exercise 1.3 requires students to go to the literature and find a peer-reviewed article using at least one principle of high reliability in a healthcare setting. Students should thoroughly read the article and be prepared to identify and define the high reliability principle presented as well as explain how the high reliability principle was applied.

These exercises can be accomplished in a discussion occurring in the physical classroom, in an online synchronous classroom, or in an facilitator-prompted course-platform-based discussion board.

STUDENT EVALUATION

Facilitators should evaluate the following:

1.1 Was the student able to give examples of current internal and external drivers that affect current healthcare organizations?

1.2 Was the student able to articulate how various applications of high reliability influence organizational approach to quality and safety at a broad and specific level?

1.3 Was the student able to explain general characteristics of high reliability principles?

CHAPTER 2

DRIVERS FOR PATIENT SAFETY

In this chapter, students will learn about the drivers for patient safety within the context of high reliability principles to better understand patient harm and its impact. Students will also learn about drivers for patient safety that relate to the individual and to shared accountability across the system of care.

Learning Objective

Summarize safety drivers affecting healthcare delivery systems and explore how HROs contribute to patient safety.

Learning Activity 2.1: Differentiate Individual and System Factors Within Patient Harm Events Through Application of High Reliability Principles to Discover Solutions and Explore Barriers

Learning Activity Objectives

2.1 Describe the multiple layers and perspectives of patient harm in an HRO (*understanding*).

2.2 Explain the interconnection of high reliability and safety culture (*applying*).

2.3 Appraise current solutions for improving safety in HROs (*analyzing*).

2.4 Consider historical and current barriers to highly reliable solutions (*evaluating*).

Preparation

Prior to completion of the learning activity, students should:

- Read Chapter 2.
- View the video *The Josie King Story* at https://www.youtube.com/watch?v=xA22_QEWapo. Consider individual and system factors that led to the error.
- Read "Human Error: Models and Management" at https://doi.org/10.1136/bmj.320.7237.768.

Instructions

2.1 Define and give two examples of latent and active failures that lead to patient harm (see Table 2.1).

Answer Example:

TABLE 2.1 LATENT AND ACTIVE FAILURES

	Definition	Examples From Your Experience
Latent failures (blunt end)	Example: Failure of oversight and support for new graduate nurses.	Example: After orientation, new nurse does not have a mentor for continued support.
Active failures (sharp end)	Example: New nurse makes an error due to lack of knowledge and fails to ask questions.	Example: Nurse makes an error in a procedure. She had never performed this procedure, did not know there was a policy, and did not know she could refuse an assignment due to lack of experience with a procedure.

2.2 Describe the Swiss cheese model of error.

- Discuss the latent factors and how they may contribute to error.
- Discuss the impact of strong and weak barriers that allow or prevent harm.

- Discuss system controls and individual controls that might strengthen barriers (block the holes in the Swiss cheese).

2.3 Find two definitions of a safety culture: Discuss solutions and barriers to achieving a safety culture based on the definitions in your current context.
- Discuss two individual factors as antidotes to patient harm.
- Discuss two system factors as antidotes to patient harm.

2.4 Present an adverse event (from experience or the literature) that led to harm.
- Apply one principle of high reliability that might have prevented the outcome.
- Discuss barriers to the principle identified.

LEARNING ACTIVITY IMPLEMENTATION

Students will benefit most from the learning activities by working individually rather than in a group.

For Exercise 2.1, facilitators should guide students to use the template provided. Facilitators should direct students to be prepared to define and give two examples of latent and active failures that lead to patient harm.

For Exercise 2.2, students should be able to describe the Swiss cheese model of error in their own words. Facilitators should guide students to reference latent factors from Exercise 2.1, the impact of strong and weak barriers that lead to or prevent harm along with system controls, and individual controls that might strengthen barriers (block the holes in the Swiss cheese).

For Exercise 2.3, facilitators should direct students to the textbook and literature to find two definitions of a safety culture. Facilitators should then guide students to discuss solutions and barriers to achieving a safety culture based on the safety culture definitions. These student discussions should be in the context of the student's current organization. In addition, facilitators should guide student discussion to include dialogue related to both individual factors and system factors as antidotes to patient harm.

For Exercise 2.4, students present an adverse event to the class. The adverse event may be an event from either student experiences or one reported in the literature. Student presentations must include application of one principle of high reliability that might have prevented the outcome along with associated barriers.

These exercises can be accomplished in a discussion occurring in the physical classroom, in an online synchronous classroom, or in a facilitator-prompted course-platform-based discussion board.

STUDENT EVALUATION

Facilitators should evaluate the following:

2.1 Was the student able to give examples of latent and active failures?

2.2 Was the student able to articulate how an error can occur and go through many layers of weak barriers prior to harming a patient?

2.3 Was the student able to define a safety culture and its characteristics?

2.4 Was the student able to articulate how an adverse event affects the individual and the workforce?

CHAPTER 3

CURRENT QUALITY DRIVERS

In this chapter, students will learn about current quality drivers for patient and healthcare outcomes. Students will also learn about high reliability as a framework for developing and sustaining a culture within healthcare organizations to provide care that minimizes errors and embraces current best evidence to achieve exceptional performance in quality, safety, and cost effectiveness.

Learning Objective

Explain current evidence-based quality drivers in the context of high reliability.

Learning Activity 3.1: Discover How Evidence-Based Practice Aligns With High Reliability Principles to Inform Drivers of Quality

Learning Activity Objectives

3.1 Describe four key drivers of current quality indicators (*remembering*).

3.2 Discuss the interrelationships between the drivers (*understanding*).

3.3 Identify two key quality nursing indicators and improvement ideas based on high reliability principles (*applying*).

Preparation

Prior to completion of the learning activity, students should:

- Read Chapter 3.
- Read "Deimplementation in Clinical Practice. What Are We Waiting For?" at https://doi.org/10.4037/aacnacc2019607.
- Read "Building Cultures of High Reliability: Lessons From the High Reliability Organization Paradigm" at https://doi.org/10.1016/j.anclin.2023.03.012.

Instructions

3.1 Select an evidence-based practice (EBP) model from the literature or your organization. Provide a short rationale for model selection and a brief overview (see Table 3.1).

Answer Example:

TABLE 3.1 EVIDENCE-BASED PRACTICE MODEL

Evidence-Based Practice Model: Iowa Model Revised: EBP to Promote Excellence in Healthcare

Rationale for Selection: Provides a structured and systematic approach to integrating research findings into clinical practice. The model aims to improve patient outcomes, enhance nursing practice and manage costs by facilitating application of evidence to clinical decisions.

Brief Overview: Iowa Model guides clinicians and organizations in translating research findings into practice, improving patient outcomes, and transforming nursing roles. The model is used by clinicians, nurses, and healthcare providers to make decisions about practice changes. The Iowa Model is a problem-solving approach that helps healthcare professionals identify, evaluate, and implement changes in practice.

Key Focus/Emphasis	Key Concepts	Steps/Stages	Strengths	Limitations
The Iowa Model helps healthcare providers implement and maintain EBP changes Focuses on the entire healthcare system, including patients, practitioners and infrastructure	Triggers to improve practice	Identify a triggering issue of opportunity: Recognize a problem or area for improvement within practice. State purpose and seek support: Define the goal of the project and ensure buy-in from relevant stakeholders. Form a team, conduct a literature review and critically appraise the evidence: Assemble a team, gather and appraise relevant evidence. Design and implement the change: Develop and implement an evidence-based practice guideline or intervention. Evaluate the change: Assess the impact of the intervention and make adjustments as needed. Disseminate the results: Share the findings and lessons learned with others.	Systematic approach Focus on frontline practice Local development and adaptability Pilot testing Emphasis on organizational support Clear steps and flow	Time-consuming Potential for delays Reliance on adequate evidence Focus on large organizations Lack of specific team composition guidelines

3.2 Identify one Nursing Quality Indicator and one Hospital Consumer Assessment of Healthcare Providers and Systems (HCAHPS) item. Include evidence from the literature supporting the quality indicator and HCAHPS item and a national benchmark for each (see Table 3.2).

Answer Example:

TABLE 3.2 NURSING QUALITY INDICATOR AND HCAHPS

Nursing Quality Indicator: Patient falls		
Indicator Definition/Description:	**Supporting Evidence/Sources:**	**National Benchmark/Benchmark Source:**
The NDNQI (National Database of Nursing Quality Indicators) defines a patient fall as an unplanned descent to the floor with or without injury to the patient. This definition includes falls where a patient lands on a surface where they shouldn't be, such as a bed or chair.	Gormley, E., Connolly, M., & Ryder, M. (2024). The development of nursing-sensitive indicators: A critical discussion. International Journal of Nursing Studies Advances, 100227.	.68 falls with injury per 1000 patient days https://www.pressganey.com/platform/ndnqi/
HCAHPS Item:		
Item Definition/Description:	**Supporting Evidence/Sources:**	**National Benchmark/Benchmark Source:**
Communication with Nurses - During this hospital stay, how often did nurses treat you with courtesy and respect? - During this hospital stay, how often did nurses listen carefully to you? - During this hospital stay, how often did nurses explain things in a way you could understand?	Kwame, A., & Petrucka, P. M. (2021). A literature-based study of patient-centered care and communication in nurse-patient interactions: barriers, facilitators, and the way forward. *BMC Nursing, 20*(1), 158.	Benchmark: 80 Source: https://hcahpsonline.org/en/

3.3 Apply the steps of an EBP model aligned with principles of high reliability to change practice (see Table 3.3).

Answer Example:

TABLE 3.3 EBP MODEL AND HIGH RELIABILITY

EBP Model: Iowa Model Revised: EBP to Promote Excellence in Healthcare	
Steps:	High Reliability Principle Alignment:
Identify a triggering issue of opportunity: Recognize a problem or area for improvement within practice.	Identifying a triggering issue aligns with **preoccupation with failure** in HROs, where teams are constantly vigilant for potential problems and risks. The Iowa Model's emphasis on identifying triggers (problem-focused or knowledge-focused) fosters this proactive approach.
State purpose and seek support: Define the goal of the project and ensure buy-in from relevant stakeholders.	Seeking support for an identified triggering issue aligns with **preoccupation with failure** in HROs, where teams are constantly vigilant for potential problems and risks. The Iowa Model's emphasis on identifying triggers (problem-focused or knowledge-focused) fosters this proactive approach.
Form a team, conduct a literature review and critically appraise the evidence: Assemble a team, gather and appraise relevant evidence.	Forming a team aligns with **deference to expertise** in HROs, where teams leverage the skills and knowledge of different members to address complex issues. The Iowa Model emphasizes collaborative decision-making, recognizing that different perspectives are crucial for effective EBP implementation.
	Conducting a literature review aligns with **sensitivity to operations** in HROs, where organizations actively monitor their systems and processes for potential problems. The literature review ensures that teams are informed about current research and best practices, enabling them to make evidence-based decisions.
	Critically appraising the evidence aligns with **reluctance to simplify** in HROs, where organizations avoid making hasty assumptions and recognize the complexity of the work they do. The critical appraisal process helps ensure that the evidence used is valid and reliable.
Design and implement the change: Develop and implement an evidence-based practice guideline or intervention.	Designing the change aligns with **commitment to resilience** in HROs, where organizations are adaptable and able to recover from unexpected events. The EBP standard provides a framework for consistent and effective implementation of the new practice.
	Implementing the change aligns with **sensitivity to operations** in HROs, where organizations constantly monitor their systems and processes for potential problems. The implementation phase involves careful planning and execution, ensuring that the new practice is integrated into the organization's workflows.
Evaluate the change: Assess the impact of the intervention and make adjustments as needed.	Evaluating the change outcome aligns with **preoccupation with failure** in HROs, where organizations are constantly vigilant for potential problems and risks. The evaluation phase provides valuable feedback on the effectiveness of the EBP standard, allowing for continuous improvement.
Disseminate the results: Share the findings and lessons learned with others.	Dissemination aligns with **sensitivity to operations** in HROs, where organizations share their knowledge and experience with others. Disseminating the results helps other organizations learn from the experience and improve their own practices.

LEARNING ACTIVITY IMPLEMENTATION

Students will benefit most from the learning activities by working in groups, but these exercises may be done individually as well.

For Exercise 3.1, facilitators should guide students to select an EBP model used by their current organization or select a model from the literature. Students should provide a short rationale for model selection as well as a brief overview of the model that includes key focus/emphasis, key concepts, steps/stages, and strengths/limitations.

For Exercise 3.2, students select one Nursing Quality Indicator and one HCAHPS item. Facilitators should guide students to retrieve evidence from the literature supporting the quality indicator and the HCAHPS item. Include a national benchmark for the quality indicator and HCAHPS item in the supporting literature.

For Exercise 3.3, facilitators should direct students to apply the steps of the selected EBP model to change practice to improve patient outcomes. The students should be able to present steps for suggested practice changes in the context of the selected EBP model that show alignment with principles of high reliability.

These exercises can be accomplished in a discussion occurring in the physical classroom, in an online synchronous classroom, or in a facilitator-prompted course-platform-based discussion board. Facilitators may consider this exercise a graded presentation.

STUDENT EVALUATION

Facilitators should evaluate the following:

3.1 Was the student able to select an EBP model? Was a rationale for selection and model overview included?

3.2 Was the student able to provide evidence supporting individual selection of one Nursing Quality Indicator and one HCAHPS item? Was a national benchmark for each included?

3.3 Was the student able to apply steps for practice changes in the context of the EBP model that show alignment with principles of high reliability?

CHAPTER 4

ORGANIZATIONAL CULTURE AND PSYCHOLOGICAL SAFETY: BREAKING DOWN BARRIERS

In this chapter, students will learn about organizational and safety culture. Students will also learn about the cultural component of psychological safety and the importance of leadership and leader actions in developing psychological safety.

Learning Objective

Examine psychological safety as a cultural component of organizational and safety culture.

Learning Activity 4.1: Compare and Contrast Facilitators and Barriers of Psychological Safety and Discuss Practical Measures of Psychological Safety

Learning Activity Objectives

4.1 Compare characteristics of a psychologically and non-psychologically safe workplace (*understanding*).

4.2 Show facilitators and barriers to psychological safety (*understanding*).

4.3 Illustrate how an organization measures psychological safety in a high reliability culture of safety (*understanding*).

Preparation

Prior to completion of the learning activity, students should:

- Read Chapter 4.
- Read "Defining and Assessing Organizational Culture" at https://doi.org/10.1111/j.1744-6198.2010.00207.x.
- Read "What Is Psychological Safety?" at https://hbr.org/2023/02/what-is-psychological-safety.

Instructions

4.1 Define and observe deep-seated assumptions and beliefs, espoused values, and artifacts of culture within your own organization.

Assumptions and beliefs: What are the driving forces behind your organization? This could be religious affiliation, for profit, not for profit, and so on. These assumptions and beliefs may be hidden, but they drive the values and artifacts of your culture.

My organization believes that . . .

Espoused values: What is the written vision or mission statement of your organization?

Our vision or mission statement is written as . . .

Artifacts: The visible manifestations of the values and beliefs of the system. This can include policies, art in the hospital, work environment, standard behaviors, expectations of leaders, reward systems, and more.

Our values are made visible by . . .

4.2 Discuss characteristics of psychological safety and non-psychological safety in the workplace. Include facilitators and barriers (see Table 4.1).

Answer Example:

TABLE 4.1 PSYCHOLOGICAL SAFETY IN THE WORKPLACE

Psychologically Safe Environment				
Event	What Happens at Your Organization?	Psychologically or Non-Psychologically Safe Workplace?	Facilitator	Barrier
I made a medication error and reported my mistake. My coworker with years of experience told me I should not have reported my error as I will get in trouble.	My director thanked me for admitting my mistake and reporting the error.	Psychologically safe: Willing to admit mistakes without fear of negative consequences.	Speaking up facilitates a psychologically safe workplace.	Dominant member of the team makes it less psychologically safe for others on the team to report errors.
Non- Psychologically Safe Environment				
Event	What Happens at Your Organization?	Psychologically or Non-Psychologically Safe Workplace?	Facilitator	Barrier
I made a medication error and reported my mistake. My coworker with years of experience told me I should not have reported my error as I will get in trouble.	My director tells me it is my fault, and I need to pay more attention to what I am doing. She puts a note in my employee file that I made a medication error.	Non-psychologically safe: Not willing to report future errors as "I will get in trouble."	Fear of speaking up facilitates a non-psychologically safe workplace.	Authoritarian or autocratic leadership style is a barrier to creating psychological safety in the workplace.

4.3 Illustrate how an organization measures psychological safety in a high reliability culture of safety in an online discussion.

- Does the organization measure psychological safety?
- Describe the measurement instrument and why it was selected.
- What are the current measures of psychological safety?
- What is the best and lowest performing category?
- How would you go about improving the scores?
- What facilitators and barriers do you see to improving scores?

LEARNING ACTIVITY IMPLEMENTATION

Students will benefit most from the learning activities by working in groups, but these exercises may be done individually as well.

For Exercise 4.1, students should thoroughly explore organizational culture and the impact to high reliability. It will be helpful to learning if students understand the concepts of organizational culture first and then apply their learning by observing their own organization.

For Exercise 4.2, students will build on Exercise 4.1 by discussing psychological safety as a cornerstone of workplace culture. Students should brainstorm how they would make psychological safety real, visible, and embedded into culture. Facilitators should guide discussion of portals and barriers to psychological safety at the individual, team, and organizational level.

For Exercise 4.3, facilitators should guide an online discussion about organizational culture, tools used to measure psychological safety, measurement results, and portals/barriers to improving scores with students. Illustrate how an organization measures psychological safety in a high reliability culture of safety in an online discussion.

These exercises can be accomplished in a discussion occurring in the physical classroom, in an online synchronous classroom, or in an instructor-prompted course-platform-based discussion board. Facilitators may consider these exercises as a graded paper or presentation.

STUDENT EVALUATION

Facilitators should evaluate the following:

4.1 Was the student able to describe how culture is created, articulated, and manifested in everyday organizational life?

4.2 Was the student able to observe and describe psychological safety, including barriers and facilitators, in the workplace?

4.3 Was the student able to describe how psychological safety culture might be assessed and changed?

CHAPTER 5

SAFETY LEADERSHIP: COMMITMENT TO HIGH RELIABILITY ORGANIZING

In this chapter, students will learn about the vital role of leadership in creating an HRO. Students will also learn about safety leadership style and associated safety leadership actions in a high reliability organizing framework to create the fearless workplace.

Learning Objective

Explain and discuss the vital role of leadership in an HRO.

Learning Activity 5.1: Compare and Contrast Characteristics of Safety Leadership Styles and Safety Leadership Actions Within a High Reliability Organizing Framework

Learning Activity Objectives

5.1 Describe the influence of different safety leadership styles and safety leadership actions on high reliability organizational quality and safety (*understanding*).

5.2 Summarize high reliability organizing as a framework for high reliability safety leadership (*understanding*).

5.3 Explain leadership strategies to build a high reliability "fearless workplace" (*applying*).

Preparation

Prior to completion of the learning activity, students should:

- Read Chapter 5.
- Read *The Fearless Organization: Creating Psychological Safety in the Workplace for Learning, Innovation, and Growth*, by Amy Edmondson.
- Consider various safety leadership styles and their influence on safety leadership actions.
- Consider the role of psychological safety in an HRO.

Instructions

5.1 Interview a local leader at your facility using the following questions and record your answers (see Table 5.1). Be prepared to share with your colleagues.

TABLE 5.1 SAFETY LEADERSHIP INTERVIEW QUESTIONS

Interview Questions	Response Notes
What events in your life have had the most positive impact on your leadership and strategic thinking development? What has had the most negative impact?	
What other events, programs, or education have had the most impact on your leadership and patient safety thinking?	
What is your most important core belief that guides the way you lead?	
How do you factor in culture, diversity, or other differences into your leadership?	

continues

TABLE 5.1 SAFETY LEADERSHIP INTERVIEW QUESTIONS (CONT.)

Interview Questions	Response Notes
How do you adapt your leadership to accommodate different age groups?	
What strategies have you used to develop a deeper sense of ownership in your followers' work and in their organization?	
How do you inspire others to achieve more than they expected?	
When you have had a significant setback at work, how did you respond? What did you learn from that setback?	
What are some of the methods you have used to foster safety thinking among peers, followers, and other leaders?	
When you look for the best candidate for a leadership role, what do you consider the most important characteristics?	

5.2 Describe the influence of their leadership style along with safety leadership actions on organizational quality and safety (see Table 5.2).

TABLE 5.2 SAFETY LEADERSHIP STYLE INFLUENCE AND ACTION

Leadership Style	Supporting Notes From Interview
Description	Transformational Leader: inspire staff to perform beyond expectations
Attributes	Idealized influence Inspirational motivation Intellectual stimulation Individual consideration
Behaviors	Role model Provide clarity Communicate a positive value-based vision for the future state of the organization and its employees Challenge team members to go beyond personal interests and focus attention on collective goals Encourage sharing of different perspectives on issues Challenge organizational norms

Leadership Style	Supporting Notes From Interview
Behaviors (cont.)	Question assumptions
	Encourage creative thinking
	Recognize unique needs and abilities of followers
	Coach and mentor
Safety leadership actions	Express satisfaction when jobs are performed safely
	Reward achievement of safety targets
	Continuous encouragement for safe working
	Maintain a safe working environment
	Suggest new ways of working more safely
	Encourage employees to openly discuss safety at work
	Talk about personal value and beliefs in the importance of safety
	Behave in a way that demonstrates commitment to safety
	Spend time to demonstrate how to work safely
	Listen to safety concerns

5.3 Go to the following link and complete the leadership assessment: https://www.mindtools.com/pages/article/leadership-style-quiz.htm

What is your leadership style? Based on your leadership style, use Table 5.3 to discuss how you would use high reliability organizing as a framework for your high reliability safety leadership style. Include specific strategies for each of the five high reliability principles that may assist you as a leader to move in the direction toward high reliability.

TABLE 5.3 MY HIGH RELIABILITY SAFETY LEADERSHIP STYLE AND STRATEGIES

High Reliability Organizing Framework	Leadership Strategies
Leadership preoccupation with failure	Articulate expectations
	Create awareness of vulnerability
	Actively track down bad news
	Clarify what constitutes good news
	Consolidate your expectations
	A near miss is a failure
Leadership reluctance to simplify	Forget some names
	Think and question out loud
	Develop skeptics
	Seek requisite variety
	Put a premium on interpersonal skills
	Revise assessments as evidence changes

continues

TABLE 5.3 MY HIGH RELIABILITY SAFETY LEADERSHIP STYLE AND STRATEGIES (CONT.)

High Reliability Organizing Framework	Leadership Strategies
Leadership sensitivity to operations	Be guided by actionable questions and structured conversations
	Cultivate situated humility
	Encourage people to simulate their work mentally
	Be physically and socially available
	Reward contact with the front line
	Speak up
	Bring unique knowledge to the surface
Leadership commitment to resilience	Adopt a mindset of cure rather than prevention
	Enlarge competencies and response repertoires
	Do not overdo Lean ideals
	Accelerate feedback
	Treat past experience with ambivalence
Leadership deference to expertise	Ask for help
	Create flexible decision structures
	Encourage imagination as a tool for managing the unexpected
	Beware of the fallacy of centrality
	Refine your grasp of expertise
	Listen with humility

5.4 As a high reliability organizing leader, apply Edmondson's three-phase leadership strategy to build a fearless organization. Include psychological safety, healthy work environment, and fearless workplace in your discussion (use Table 5.4 to record your responses).

TABLE 5.4 THREE-PHASE LEADERSHIP STRATEGY

Leadership Strategy Phase	Leadership Strategies
Phase I: Setting the Stage	Articulate how employee jobs are interdependent
	Articulate how employee jobs contribute to organizational purpose
	Reframe failure as an opportunity to learn rather than an opportunity to blame

Leadership Strategy Phase	Leadership Strategies
Phase II: Inviting Participation	Be crystal clear in the invitation to participate
	Demonstrate situational humility
	Practice proactive inquiry
Phase III: Responding Appropriately	Express appreciation
	Destigmatize failure
	Sanction clear violations

LEARNING ACTIVITY IMPLEMENTATION

Students will benefit most from the learning activities when they do them individually rather than in a group.

For Exercise 5.1, students will select a leader at their current organization to interview. Students should be able to determine their leader's leadership style following the interview.

For Exercise 5.2, students should be able to discuss safety leadership style and associated safety leadership actions of the leader interviewed. Facilitators should guide students to include discussion about specific leadership style incorporating attributes, behaviors and associated safety leadership actions.

For Exercise 5.3, students should be able to discuss how high reliability organizing provides a framework for high reliability safety leadership. Facilitators should guide students to include discussion about specific safety leadership strategies with real-world examples for each of the five principles of high reliability.

For Exercise 5.4, a thorough discussion of the role of psychological safety is needed. Students should complete this exercise through the lens of a high reliability organizing leader. Students should apply Edmondson's three-phase leadership strategy to build their own fearless organization, including specific leadership strategies in each phase.

These exercises can be accomplished in a discussion occurring in the physical classroom, in an online synchronous classroom, or in a facilitator-prompted course-platform-based discussion board. Facilitators may consider these exercises as a graded paper or presentation.

STUDENT EVALUATION

Facilitators should evaluate the following:

5.1 Was the student able to interview a leader at their organization and determine their leadership style?

5.2 Was the student able to describe the influence of a specific safety leadership style and safety leadership actions on high reliability organizational quality and safety?

5.3 Was the student able to review high reliability organizing as a framework for high reliability safety leadership?

5.4 Was the student able to articulate specific leadership strategies that could be applied to build a highly reliable fearless organization?

CHAPTER 6

HEALTH EQUITY AND HIGH RELIABILITY: CONNECTING THE DOTS FOR PATIENT SAFETY

In this chapter, students will learn about the relationship between health equity and high reliability. Students will also learn how to incorporate health equity concepts into patient safety and quality work.

Learning Objective

Explain how combining health equity and high reliability principles makes patient safety and quality work meaningful for patient populations.

Learning Activity 6.1: Use Health Equity Knowledge to Inform Patient Safety Initiatives

Learning Activity Objectives

6.1 Relate ethical frameworks to provide equitable care (*understanding*).

6.2 Articulate ways to address challenges in promoting equitable care (*applying*).

6.3 Defend the importance of addressing root causes of health disparities as a way to promote patient safety (*evaluating*).

6.4 Compile the links between health equity and HRO principles (*creating*).

Preparation

Prior to completion of the learning activity, students should:

- Read Chapter 6
- Read "From HRO to HERO: Making Health Equity a Core System Capability" at https://doi.org/10.1097/JMQ.0000000000000020.

Instructions

6.1 Select one of the following ethical frameworks or approaches for decision-making and write one or two paragraphs explaining why the selected framework compels actions that promote health equity. Resource: https://www.pbs.org/wnet/religionandethics/files/2008/09/five_sources.pdf.
   - Utilitarianism
   - Rights-based ethics
   - Fairness and justice approach
   - The common good approach
   - Virtue ethics

6.2 Create a one-page SBAR to explain the concern, give some background, and provide an assessment and recommendations for the following situation.

   You received a complaint from a Latinx patient who states the hospital staff was disrespectful and provided biased care because he is an immigrant. He was not offered interpretation and was made to wait in the ED waiting room longer than other people who came in after him. The patient believes he received poor treatment because in the current political climate immigrants are not welcomed. You want to communicate this to your supervisor and make recommendations that will support both staff and community members.

6.3 You have been asked to do an interview where you will defend the following premise: Addressing the root causes of health disparities is important for sustaining health equity work and for patient safety.

Record yourself answering the following interview questions:

- What are the root causes of health disparities?

- Can you speak to one specific patient, provider, system, or social factor that is at the root of health disparities and tell us why it is important to address it and share best practices for addressing it?

- Why is addressing the root causes of health disparities, like discrimination, essential to patient safety?

6.4 Reflect on the links between health equity and high reliability principles to complete the following statements:

- When looking at health equity, *preoccupation with failure* means:

- I can demonstrate *reluctance to simply* when addressing health disparities by:

- One way to practice the principle of *sensitivity to operations* when looking at existing disparities within a system is:

- HROs can demonstrate *deference to expertise* by:

- *Commitment to resilience* related to health equity is evident in an organization when:

LEARNING ACTIVITY IMPLEMENTATION

Students will benefit most from the learning activities by working individually.

For Exercise 6.1, students will select an ethical framework or approach to decision-making and write one or two paragraphs that explain why the ethical framework/decision-making model was selected. Students should be able to explain why the selected ethical framework/decision-making model compels actions that promote health equity.

For Exercise 6.2, students should be able to create an SBAR for the hypothetical situation. Students should articulate ways to address challenges in promoting equitable care.

For Exercise 6.3, students should be able to defend the importance of addressing root causes of health disparities to promote patient safety. Students should articulate the connection between root causes of health disparities, health equity work, and patient safety.

For Exercise 6.4, students should be able to link health equity and HRO principles. Students should apply all HRO principles to health equity concepts.

These exercises can be accomplished in a discussion occurring in the physical classroom, in an online synchronous classroom, or in a facilitator-prompted course-platform-based discussion board. Facilitators may consider these exercises as a graded paper or presentation.

STUDENT EVALUATION

Facilitators should evaluate the following:

6.1 Was the student able to select an ethical framework/decision-making model and explain why the ethical framework/decision-making model compels actions that promote health equity?

6.2 Was the student able to create an SBAR to address challenges in promoting equitable care?

6.3 Was the student able to defend the importance of addressing root causes of health disparities to sustain health equity work to promote patient safety?

6.4 Was the student able to link HRO principles with health equity concepts?

PART II

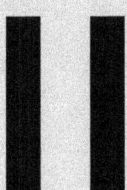

HRO CONCEPTS AND APPLICATION TO PRACTICE: PREOCCUPATION WITH FAILURE

Learning Objective

Recommend quality and safety activities based on high reliability principles (*evaluating*).

Contents

Chapter 7   Using Failure Mode and Effects Analysis to Predict Failure 42

Chapter 8   Paying Attention to Close Calls and Near Misses 46

CHAPTER 7

USING FAILURE MODE AND EFFECTS ANALYSIS TO PREDICT FAILURE

In this chapter, students will learn about anticipation of failure in an HRO. Students will also learn about the purpose, potential uses, and challenges of completing a Failure Mode and Effects Analysis (FMEA).

Learning Objective

Explain and discuss the vital role of anticipation of failure in an HRO.

Learning Activity 7.1: Discuss the Importance of the FMEA Process Within a High Reliability Organization

Learning Activity Objectives

7.1 Describe the use of the FMEA as a cornerstone of high reliability (*understanding*).

7.2 Discuss various applications of the FMEA in healthcare (*understanding*).

7.3 Apply concepts of the FMEA to explore potential failures within practice (*applying*).

Preparation

Prior to completion of the learning activity, students should:

- Read Chapter 7.
- Search the literature and find and read one article that uses FMEA as an improvement method.
- Review "Guidance for Performing Failure Mode and Effects Analysis With Performance Improvement Projects" at https://www.cms.gov/Medicare/Provider-Enrollment-and-Certification/QAPI/Downloads/GuidanceForFMEA.pdf.
- Read "Systems Thinking, Culture of Reliability and Safety" at https://www.icesi.edu.co/blogs/pslunes122/files/2012/08/Systems-thinking-culture-of-reliability-and-safety1.pdf.
- Think about the concept of safety imagination and how safety imagination is a key process for high reliability.

Instructions

7.1 List at least four possible opportunities to use FMEA within your practice setting. Discuss why you believe the process is right for an FMEA, including the high-risk nature of the process and the potential for failures. Who would you involve?

_____

_____

_____

_____

7.2 Within your facility, find applications of the FMEA process and list the process examined, failures found, and solutions suggested (see Table 7.1). If your facility has not completed an FMEA, use the article found in the literature as your source.

Answer Example:

TABLE 7.1 APPLYING THE FMEA PROCESS

Process Examined	Main Failure Modes	Solutions Suggested	Positive Impact of the FMEA on the Process
Examples: Medication administration	Wrong dose Missed dose Incorrect patient Failure to scan	Implement barcode scanning Double check pump guardrails Medication timeouts	Reduced medication errors and improved patient safety

7.3 Practice brainstorming failure modes: Select a common process and select one step in the process. List all the ways that the step could fail, the effect of the failure, and the reason for the failure.

Answers:

- Human failures:
    - Skill-based: Lapse, slips
    - Rule-based: Not following or applying a rule correctly
    - Knowledge-based: Guessing when entering an unfamiliar area

- System failures:
    - Poor design
    - Flawed equipment
    - Cumbersome procedures
    - Poor oversight

Answer Example:

Process: Setting alarm to wake up in the morning on time

Step to examine: Setting your alarm (see Table 7.2)

TABLE 7.2 FAILURE MODES EXAMPLE

How Could This Step Fail?	What Would Happen to the Patient or System if the Step Failed?	Why Would This Step Fail? (Describe the human or system reason.)
Forget to set the alarm	You do not get up on time.	Too tired to remember
Set the alarm for p.m. and not a.m.	You do not get up on time.	Distracted; did not double-check; did not read instructions; did not know how to set the alarm and guessed incorrectly
		Setting confusing and not easily visible

How Could This Step Fail?	What Would Happen to the Patient or System if the Step Failed?	Why Would This Step Fail? (Describe the human or system reason.)
Set time setting instead of alarm	You do not get up on time.	Distracted; did not double-check; did not read instructions; did not know how to set the alarm and guessed incorrectly
		Setting confusing and not easily visible

    7.4 Discuss the importance of psychological safety when brainstorming failure modes within a group.

LEARNING ACTIVITY IMPLEMENTATION

Students will benefit most from the learning activities by working both individually and in a group.

For Exercise 7.1, students will benefit most if they can relate the use of the FMEA tool to anticipate failures. Examination of a journal article is helpful; however, discussing how the FMEA is used within the students' own practice area will be the most valuable. Facilitators may consider this exercise as a graded paper.

For Exercise 7.2, students should find an application of the FMEA process at their organization. Facilitators should coach students to list the process examined, failures found, and solutions suggested. If students' facilities have not completed an FMEA, the students may use the article from literature in Exercise 7.1.

For Exercise 7.3, students will benefit most working in a group to brainstorm. Brainstorming failure modes and seeking worst-case scenarios is not routine for most healthcare providers. We usually do not want to focus on how we can fail. Sharing how students' own experience with identifying failure modes in existing processes before they cause harm would be a good discussion forum.

For Exercise 7.4, students build on Exercise 7.3 to include a discussion of the importance of psychological safety when brainstorming failure modes.

These exercises can be accomplished in a discussion occurring in the physical classroom, in an online synchronous classroom, or in an facilitator-prompted course-platform-based discussion board. Facilitators may consider these exercises as a graded paper or a presentation.

STUDENT EVALUATION

Facilitators should evaluate the following:

    7.1 Was the student able to understand the relationship between use of the FMEA and anticipation of failure?

    7.2 Was the student able to articulate the impact to organizational safety when an FMEA is used?

    7.3 Was the student able to list opportunities for use of the FMEA?

    7.4 Was the student able to apply brainstorming for failure modes within a process?

CHAPTER 8

PAYING ATTENTION TO CLOSE CALLS AND NEAR MISSES

In this chapter, students will learn about why reporting close calls, near misses, and unsafe conditions is the best opportunity to anticipate and fix failures before harm is caused to a patient or system.

Learning Objective

Discuss how the identification and mitigation of near misses, close calls, and unsafe conditions promotes high reliability.

Learning Activity 8.1: Evaluate the Importance of Near Misses, Close Calls, and Unsafe Conditions to High Reliability

Learning Activity Objectives

8.1 Define near miss, close call, and unsafe condition (*remembering*).

8.2 Describe the importance of identifying near misses and close calls to improve safety (*understanding*).

8.3 Discuss barriers to reporting and acting on near misses and close calls within the current environment (*understanding*).

Preparation

Prior to completion of the learning activity, students should do:

- Read Chapter 8.
- Read "Nurses' Experiences in Voluntary Error Reporting: An Integrative Literature Review" at https://doi.org/10.1016/j.ijnss.2021.07.004.
- Read "Reporting and Responding to Patient Safety Incidents Based on Data From Hospitals' Reporting Systems: A Systematic Review" at https://doi.org/10.5430/jha.v9n2p22.

Instructions

8.1 Ask three coworkers to identify a recent near miss, close call, or unsafe condition that they think might lead to patient harm in the near future.

- Ask if they have reported the issue through a formal reporting system. Why or why not?
- What was done to remedy the situation?
- Ask if they are currently aware of "workarounds" to get things done.
- Do they consider the "workaround" an issue worth reporting?

8.2 Discuss barriers and facilitators to reporting near misses, close calls, or unsafe conditions.

8.3 Discuss three strategies to make reporting events easier and more useful to improve patient safety.

LEARNING ACTIVITY IMPLEMENTATION

Students will benefit most from the learning activities by working individually rather than in a group.

For Exercise 8.1, students will ask three coworkers about a recent near miss, close call, or unsafe condition. Facilitators should guide students to think about how these events might lead to patient harm. Students will benefit most from this exercise if they can discuss real-life experiences of healthcare staff in identifying and reporting near misses, close calls, and unsafe situations.

For Exercise 8.2, students should discuss barriers and facilitators of reporting near misses, close calls, or unsafe conditions. Facilitators should guide students to discuss experiences from their organizations.

For Exercise 8.3, students build on Exercise 8.2 to discuss three strategies to mitigate barriers to make reporting events easier. Facilitators should coach students to include discussion on how the strategies could be useful to staff to improve patient safety.

These exercises can be accomplished in a discussion occurring in the physical classroom, in an online synchronous classroom, or in a facilitator-prompted course-platform-based discussion board. Facilitators could also assign these exercises as a graded paper or a presentation.

STUDENT EVALUATION

Facilitators should evaluate the following:

8.1 Was the student able to discuss the value of reporting near misses and close calls? Was the student able to identify significant near misses, close calls, unsafe conditions, and workarounds? Was the student able to discuss how the identification of these events can improve patient safety?

8.2 Was the student able to summarize barriers and facilitators of reporting near misses, close calls, and unsafe conditions?

8.3 Was the student able to discuss ways to make reporting events easier to improve patient safety?

PART III

HRO CONCEPTS AND APPLICATION TO PRACTICE: RELUCTANCE TO SIMPLIFY

Learning Objective

Recommend quality and safety activities based on high reliability principles (*evaluating*).

Contents

Chapter 9   Human Factors Engineering for Reducing and
            Recovering From Error 50

Chapter 10 Root Cause Analysis: A Tool for High Reliability in
            a Complex Environment 55

Chapter 11 Fostering Just Culture in High Reliability Organizations:
            How Far Have We Come? 59

CHAPTER 9

HUMAN FACTORS ENGINEERING FOR REDUCING AND RECOVERING FROM ERROR

In this chapter, students will learn about the scope and practice of human factors engineering (HFE). Students will also learn about the value of partnering with trained HFE practitioners in their efforts to improve patient safety as well as the safety of those on the front lines of healthcare.

Learning Objective

Explore the value of HFE to improve the safety of patients and clinicians.

Learning Activity 9.1: Explain Human Factors Engineering (HFE): The Science and Practice of Designing Work Systems to Fit the Needs, Limitations, and Capabilities of Humans

Learning Activity Objectives

9.1 Discuss how practitioners of HFE think about work systems (*understanding*).

9.2 Explain how the design of the work system can make it easier for errors to occur and harder to recover from (*applying*).

9.3 Explain how practitioners of HFE approach redesigning the work system to reduce opportunities for error and to facilitate recovery from error (*analyzing*).

Preparation

Prior to completion of the learning activity, students should:

- Read Chapter 9.
- Read "SEIPS 2.0: A Human Factors Framework for Studying and Improving the Work of Healthcare Professionals and Patients" at https://doi.org/10.1080/00140139.2013.838643.
- Read "Process Mapping—The Foundation for Effective Quality Improvement" at https://doi.org/10.1016/j.cppeds.2018.08.010.

Instructions

9.1 Identify an error-prone process for improvement at your organization.

9.2 Form a group to map out the current process targeted for improvement.

9.3 Identify the characteristics of work system elements (persons, tools/technology, tasks, physical environment, and organizational environment) that make it easier/harder for errors to happen. Include learning from error in your discussion.

Answer Example:

Table 9.1 shows an example of responding to an emergent situation occurring in a negative pressure air flow room that requires responders to quickly don full personal protective equipment (PPE).

TABLE 9.1 ERROR-PRONE PROCESS FOR IMPROVEMENT

Work System Element Characteristics (persons, tools/technology, tasks, physical environment, organizational environment)	Easier for Errors to Happen? Why?	Harder for Errors to Happen? Why?	Learning From Error
Physical availability of PPE	If PPE is not available and has to be searched for, a delay in care will occur.	Ensure that the required PPE is stocked outside of the room.	A simulation of responding to an emergent situation for a patient in an isolation room would be an example of practicing and learning from error before the error harms a patient.
Direction on "which" PPE should be used	If the type of PPE required for the patient is not specified, a delay will occur.	Ensure that a list for the PPE required is on the door of the patient room.	
Ease of "donning" PPE	If PPE is too difficult to "don," a delay in care will occur.	Practice "donning" PPE in an emergent situation.	

9.4 Brainstorm corrective actions that target/leverage these characteristics and do not rely heavily on things like training, instructions for use, and warnings to work (see Table 9.2).

Answer Example:

TABLE 9.2 CORRECTIVE ACTIONS BRAINSTORMING

Work Element Characteristic	Corrective Action
Donning PPE	Simulation donning PPE
Availability of PPE	Simulate inventory management systems
	Conserve PPE usage (prioritize PPE use, bundle patient care activities)
	Waste reduction (PPE usage patterns)
Which PPE to use	Hazard assessment (identify risks, evaluate risks)

9.5 Discuss the types of human errors that most commonly occur. Give examples and a possible solution from a human factor's perspective (see Table 9.3 for an example).

Answer Example:

TABLE 9.3 TYPES OF HUMAN FACTOR ERRORS

Type of Human Factor Error	Definition	Example	HFE Solution
Skill-based error	Lapse or slip during a frequently performed task, usually due to distraction or rushing	Entering order on the wrong patient	System does not allow for two patient charts to be open at the same time
Rule-based error	Applying the wrong rule, applying a rule incorrectly, or not using a known rule	Not checking renal status prior to giving a medication that may damage kidneys	Flags in medication administration system that remind to check renal status
Knowledge-based error	Guessing and not asking for help in a situation for which the person involved has no context or experience	If a patient has decreased mentation, guessing that she is just tired	Accepted triggers that mandate a call for a second opinion

LEARNING ACTIVITY IMPLEMENTATION

Students will benefit most from the learning activities by working in a group.

For Exercise 9.1, students should identify an error-prone process for improvement from their organization.

For Exercise 9.2, students build on Exercise 9.1 to form a group to identify an error-prone process for improvement from one group member's organization. Facilitators should guide each group of students to map out the current process targeted for improvement and identify characteristics of the work system elements that make errors easier or harder to happen. Facilitators should coach student groups about learning from error.

For Exercise 9.3, students brainstorm characteristics of work system elements (persons, tools/technology, tasks, physical environment, and organizational environment) that make it easier or harder for errors to happen based on their findings in Exercises 9.1 and 9.2.

For Exercise 9.4, student groups brainstorm potential corrective actions based on their findings in Exercises 9.1, 9.2, and 9.3. Students should include in their discussion human factors and ergonomics design cycle as well as how HFEs think about work systems.

For Exercise 9.5, students should identify examples of human error from their experience to better understand the types of human errors that can occur.

These exercises can be accomplished in a discussion occurring in the physical classroom, in an online synchronous classroom, or in a facilitator-prompted course-platform-based discussion board. Facilitators may consider these exercises as a graded paper or a presentation.

STUDENT EVALUATION

Facilitators should evaluate the following:

9.1 Was the student able to discuss how HFEs think about work systems?

9.2 Was the student able to explain how the design of the work system can make it easier for errors to occur and harder to recover from?

9.3 Was the student able to explain HFE's approach to redesigning the work system to reduce opportunities for error and to facilitate recovery from error?

9.4 Was the student able to suggest potential corrective actions?

9.5 Was the student able to identify examples of different types of human error?

CHAPTER 10

ROOT CAUSE ANALYSIS: A TOOL FOR HIGH RELIABILITY IN A COMPLEX ENVIRONMENT

In this chapter, students will learn about the background, processes, and challenges of using root cause analysis (RCA) as a tool to advance safety in an HRO. Students will also learn the steps in an effective RCA.

Learning Objective

Explore the usefulness and challenges of using RCA as a tool to advance safety in an HRO.

Learning Activity 10.1: Discuss Use of RCA as a Tool for Embedding the High Reliability Principle "Reluctance to Simplify" Into a Safety Event Investigation

Learning Activity Objectives

10.1 Discuss the significance of using RCA as a tool to discover system issues (*understanding*).

10.2 Apply the "Five Whys" questioning technique to a familiar problem (*applying*).

10.3 Discuss common problems that may lessen RCA effectiveness (*understanding*).

10.4 Explain how bias occurs and how to avoid bias during the RCA process (*understanding*).

Preparation

Prior to completion of the learning activity, students should:

- Read Chapter 10.
- Read "RCA²: Improving Root Cause Analysis and Actions to Prevent Harm" at https://www.med.unc.edu/ihqi/files/2018/07/RCA2-National-Patient-Safety-Foundation.pdf.

Instructions

10.1 Read the case examples regarding the errors in the first few pages of the chapter. Identify the active errors and the latent errors in the mistake (see Table 10.1).

   Answer Example:

TABLE 10.1 ACTIVE AND LATENT ERRORS

	Active Error (human error)	Latent Error (system issues)
Medication error: Antibiotic given too quickly	Nurse overrode the soft limit and did not double check the timing requirement of the antibiotic.	An error in the pharmacy printing system led to a label that had the incorrect time requirement. The nurse was following the label instructions.
Ordering error: Two patients received incorrect radiology tests	Physician rushing, mixed up two patients and ordered incorrect tests for both.	Culture focused on "production pressure": Doing things faster is rewarded and an overriding priority
Medication error: Gave insulin instead of antibiotic	Not checking the medication prior to hanging Multitasking	High risk medication not clearly identified by labeling Workload demands encourage multitasking

10.2 Discuss the impact to high reliability when system issues are identified and corrected rather than correcting the individual only. Reflect on a time in your career when an individual was blamed/disciplined for an event. How did that affect the overall culture of safety? Did the error recur?

10.3 Identify a safety issue: Practice asking "Five Whys" to get to the root cause (see Figure 10.1). The first "why" addresses the one most proximate to the error, usually a clinician. The last "why" question should be at the system level.

Answer Example:

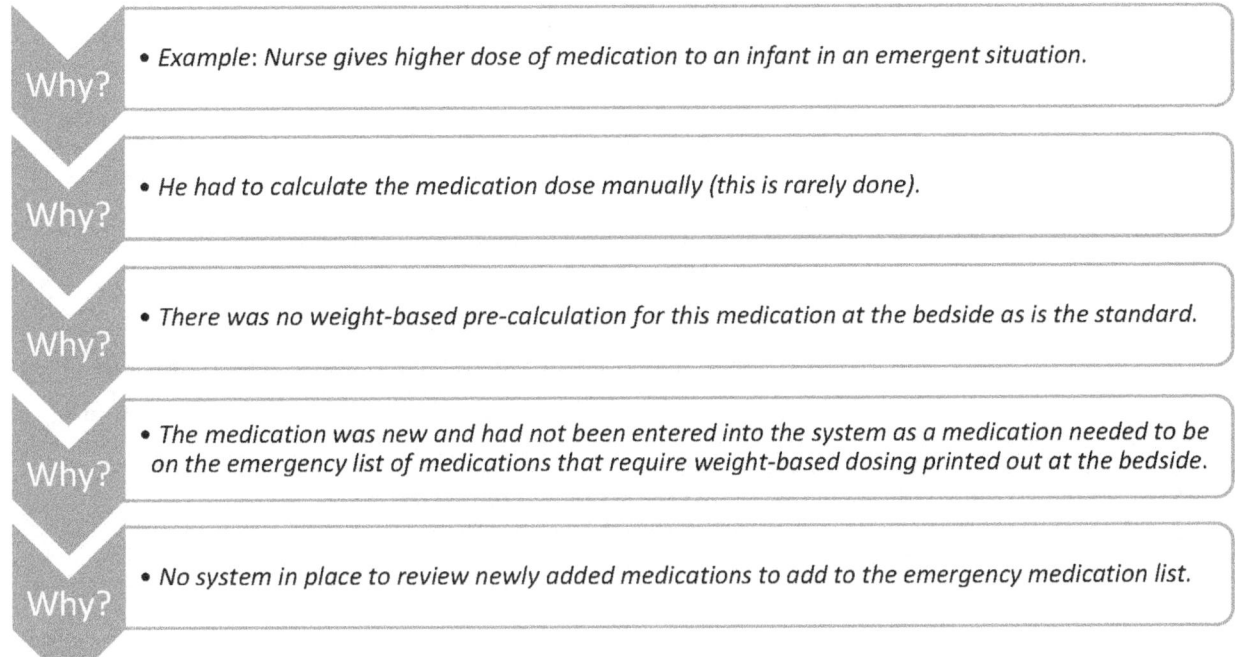

Figure 10.1 Practicing the Five Whys to get to the root cause.

10.4 List three strategies to ensure RCA is effective to prevent future error.

LEARNING ACTIVITY IMPLEMENTATION

Students will benefit most from the learning activities by working either individually or in a group.

For Exercise 10.1, students should read and reflect on the science and philosophy behind RCA and the relevance to the HRO principle of reluctance to simplify. Facilitators should guide discussion of the case examples to distinguish between the symptoms of a problem (active failures) and the root causes of a problem (latent failures). Facilitators can use the Swiss cheese model to illustrate the difference between the two types of failures.

For Exercise 10.2, students should reflect on the impact to high reliability when system issues are identified and corrected rather than correcting only the individual. Facilitators should guide discussion to include the impact of blame on the culture of safety.

For Exercise 10.3, students practice asking the "Five Whys" to the root cause of an occurrence. Facilitators should guide students to begin with the first "why" most proximate to the error and finish with a fifth "why" at the system level.

For Exercise 10.4, students list strategies to ensure RCA is effective. Facilitators should guide students to refer to the "RCA²" reading. The reading lists specific skills needed for an RCA and factors that make an RCA less effective. Students may reflect on this reading, discuss RCAs that did not make an impact and those that did. Discussion surrounding the strength of interventions used within an RCA may also be effective for learning.

These exercises can be accomplished in a discussion occurring in the physical classroom, in an online synchronous classroom, or in an facilitator-prompted course-platform-based discussion board. Facilitators may consider these exercises as a graded paper or a presentation.

STUDENT EVALUATION

Facilitators should evaluate the following:

10.1 Was the student able to articulate the difference between active and latent factors and give examples of both?

10.2 Was the student able to distinguish the significance of digging deeper than the manifest symptoms of a safety problem?

10.3 Was the student able to discuss how RCAs can be made more effective?

10.4 Was the student able to practice asking "why" until getting to a root cause?

CHAPTER 11

FOSTERING JUST CULTURE IN HIGH RELIABILITY ORGANIZATIONS: HOW FAR HAVE WE COME?

In this chapter, students will learn about Just Culture. Students will also learn about the challenges of Just Culture in practice due to outcome bias, misapplication of assumptions, and application of the Just Culture algorithm without a clear commitment to the tenets of the culture change needed to learn from errors.

Learning Objective

Discover the history, theory, and challenges of implementing Just Culture in practice.

Learning Activity 11.1: Examine the Features and Challenges of a Just Culture Within a Highly Reliable Safety Program and the Current Healthcare Environment

Learning Activity Objectives

11.1 Compare and contrast a Just Culture versus a blameless culture versus a punitive culture (*analyzing*).

11.2 Apply Just Culture principles to examples (*applying*).

11.3 Discuss challenges to a Just Culture (*understanding*).

11.4 Describe the differences between a retributive Just Culture and a restorative Just Culture (*understanding*).

11.5 Discuss the challenge of Just Culture when the patient outcome is "bad" (*applying*).

Preparation

Prior to completion of the learning activity, students should do:

- Read Chapter 11.
- Watch the video *Annie's Story* at https://youtu.be/zeldVu-3DpM.
- Find and read an article on second victim syndrome. Option: "Second Victims in Health Care: Current Perspectives" at https://doi.org/10.2147/AMEP.S185912.
- Read "Restorative Just Culture Checklist" at https://safetydifferently.com/restorative-just-culture-checklist/restorativejustculturechecklist-2/.
- Read "Reckless Homicide at Vanderbilt? A Just Culture Analysis" at https://www.linkedin.com/pulse/reckless-homicide-vanderbilt-just-culture-analysis-david-marx/.

Instructions

11.1 Discuss the differences between a blameless culture, a punitive culture, and a Just Culture and the effects to patient safety for each type of culture.

11.2 Define the three types of errors that can occur and give examples from your experience (see Table 11.1).

Answer Example:

TABLE 11.1 EXAMPLE OF DEFINING THE THREE TYPES OF ERRORS

	Definition	Example in Practice	How Is This Normally Dealt With?	How Could It Be Dealt With to Promote a Just Culture?
Human error	Example: Slips, lapses; not intentional; usually related to distraction	Getting called out of a room for an emergency and forgetting to set the bed alarm for a high-risk fall patient	Not noticed unless there is an event. Blame if there is an event	Consoling: oversight due to an emergency. Assess for "second victim"
Risky behavior	Not following a rule without realizing the significance to safety	Not turning on a bed alarm for a high-risk fall patient because the family said they would watch the patient	Blame and criticism	Coaching on the decision, retraining. Follow up with positive reinforcement
Reckless behavior	Not following a rule without regard for the significance to safety	Not turning on a bed alarm for a high-risk fall patient because the staff member is "tired of hearing the alarm"	Not noticed if no event. Disciplinary action if warranted	Assess for malicious action or impairment. Hold employee accountable with retraining/disciplinary action and immediate evidence of change

11.3 Interview a manager within your organization. Find out the following:
- Current Just Culture algorithm used in the facility
- How the manager was trained to use the algorithm
- Example of how the algorithm has been used to promote positive learning
- Whether there is a second victim program or a support system for those involved in errors
- Any difficulties in applying the Just Culture process, especially when the outcome of the error was serious

11.4 Discuss the impact of involvement in an error on the healthcare provider. Describe second victim syndrome and the effect on the individual and the healthcare system. Discuss how a restorative Just Culture can assist in healing the individual involved in the error and can affect system safety and healing.

11.5 Discuss challenges to Just Culture and outcome bias when the outcome is catastrophic. Reflect on the Vanderbilt case above or another case involving litigation or media coverage. How does the outcome bias affect the application of Just Culture?

CASE STUDY

The hospital has a new program aimed at reducing surgical site infections. The responsibility for administering antibiotics has been put in the hands of the anesthesia provider in the operating room to guarantee infusion within one hour of incision. If the patient needs a special antibiotic protocol requiring more than one antibiotic, the process is started in the pre-op area.

Kathy is an experienced pre-op nurse. A full schedule coupled with a sick call has made for a busy morning. In reviewing the schedule and her assignment, she sees that Mr. Wright is scheduled for a new procedure and will need three antibiotics before surgery. After her initial assessment, Kathy hangs the first antibiotic, Vancomycin 1 GM, and signs the medication administration sheet. She returns in 90 minutes and hangs the second antibiotic, Gentamycin 80 mg.

The CRNA, who is new to the service, stops in the pre-op area to read the chart of the patient. The CRNA takes the paper record to the conference room. Kathy returns to the bedside and checks her order on the CPOE for the final antibiotic and hangs the Ancef, 1 GM. The paper MAR is with the chart, so she makes a mental note to sign the MAR before the patient goes to the OR. The antibiotic infusion is finished, but Kathy forgets to go back to the chart because her usual practice is to sign the MAR when she hangs the medication.

An orderly comes to pick up the patient for the OR. Upon entering the OR, the CRNA notices that two of the three antibiotics have been administered and proceeds to hang Ancef prior to the procedure. The patient receives the duplicate dose before the presurgical nurse (Kathy) remembers she did not sign the MAR and calls into the room. The patient had no adverse outcome.

Questions for Discussion

1. Is this error an example of human error, negligence, recklessness, or an intentional rule violation? Support your answer with your rationale.
2. How should the unit manager approach Kathy when beginning her investigation into the situation?
3. What type of investigation would be the most effective in this situation?
4. What type of action is warranted based on the type of behavior that was displayed?

LEARNING ACTIVITY IMPLEMENTATION

Students will benefit most from the learning activities by working individually.

For Exercise 11.1, students should be able to differentiate blameless culture, punitive culture, and Just Culture. In addition, facilitators should coach students to discuss the effects of each type of culture to patient safety.

For Exercise 11.2, students should provide examples of the three types of error from practice. Facilitators should be mindful that examples from practice are helpful to understand the specific behaviors that are looked at within an error.

For Exercise 11.3, facilitators may facilitate student discussion to compare different types of Just Culture algorithms and associated variations in practice.

For Exercise 11.4, facilitators should facilitate discussion about the impact of involvement in an error on a healthcare provider. Discussion should include second victim syndrome and restorative Just Culture. This exercise could be a short, graded paper with sources of evidence.

For Exercise 11.5, facilitators should facilitate student reflection discussion on the Vanderbilt Just Culture analysis case. The role of media coverage, litigation, and outcome bias should also be included in the discussion.

The case study is optional and can be used as an online posting.

These exercises can be accomplished in a discussion occurring in the physical classroom, in an online synchronous classroom, or in a facilitator-prompted course-platform-based discussion board.

STUDENT EVALUATION

Facilitators should evaluate the following:

11.1 Was the student able to articulate the main principles of Just Culture in theory?

11.2 Was the student able to apply these principles in current practice and give examples?

11.3 Was the student able to articulate the impact of second victim syndrome and relate a restorative Just Culture to this syndrome?

11.4 Was the student able to discuss challenges to Just Culture, particularly outcome bias?

11.5 Was the student able to discuss Just Culture and the principles of high reliability in the context of the case study?

PART IV

HRO CONCEPTS AND APPLICATION TO PRACTICE: SENSITIVITY TO OPERATIONS

Learning Objective

Recommend quality and safety activities based on high reliability principles (*evaluating*).

Contents

Chapter 12 Alarm Safety: Working Solutions 65

Chapter 13 Innovative Technology, Standardization, and the Impact on High Reliability 68

Chapter 14 Tiered Safety Huddles 73

CHAPTER 12

ALARM SAFETY: WORKING SOLUTIONS

In this chapter, students will learn about improvements directed toward alarm safety in response to harm related to alarm fatigue, increased technology, and regulatory guidance. Students will also learn about interventions based on high reliability principles as a strategy for sustainable alarm safety.

Learning Objective

Explore the high-risk nature of clinical alarm management and the challenges of identifying and containing the risk to prevent adverse events.

Learning Activity 12.1: Appraise the Concept of Alarm Fatigue and the Possibilities for Improvement When Applying High Reliability Principles to Clinical Alarm Safety

Learning Activity Objectives

12.1 Consider the implications of alarm fatigue within the clinical environment (*understanding*).

12.2 Apply concepts of failure mode effects analysis (FMEA) to appraise clinical alarms within a practice environment (*applying*).

Preparation

Prior to completion of the learning activity, students should:

- Read Chapter 12.
- Read "A Call to Alarms: Current State and Future Directions in the Battle Against Alarm Fatigue" at https://www.ncbi.nlm.nih.gov/pmc/articles/PMC6263784/pdf/nihms-1502834.pdf.

Instructions

12.1 In a 500-word essay, define alarm fatigue, give examples, and discuss the implications for patient safety and high reliability.

- Include examples of actionable versus nonactionable alarms and the implication for alarm fatigue.
- Describe how healthcare organizations are improving the safety of clinical alarms.
- Discuss how these organizations use data to track progress.
- Finally, discuss how high reliability principles and improvement concepts were used in the improvement efforts.
    - Include preoccupation with failure, attention to detail, and deference to expertise.
    - Include standardization and situational awareness.

12.2 Perform an assessment of clinical alarms or noise distraction in your area of experience within an FMEA format using Table 12.1 to record your answers.

Answer Example:

TABLE 12.1 FMEA ANALYSIS OF A CLINICAL ALARM OR NOISE DISTRACTION

Alarm	Expected Response	How Could Response Fail?	What Would Happen to a Patient Due to a Failure?	Why Would This Response Fail?
Example: Low or high heart rate alarm	Clinician goes to room and checks patient immediately	Clinician does not hear alarm or is not alerted to alarm	Mortality/morbidity	Alarm volume not checked
		Clinician is in another room		No alert system
		Clinician thinks the alarm is not "real" due to frequency of false alarms		Alarm fatigue

LEARNING ACTIVITY IMPLEMENTATION

Students will benefit the most from the learning activities by working individually.

For Exercise 12.1, facilitators should guide students to define alarm fatigue, give examples, and discuss the implications for patient safety and high reliability. Students should be encouraged to go to the literature to find evidence in support of definitions and examples. This exercise could be completed as a short, graded paper with references from current literature.

For Exercise 12.2, students integrate the FMEA process into alarm assessment and safety. Students can refer to Chapter 7 in the textbook for a template or use the table provided. Students who are not in an environment with clinical alarms can interview a colleague who works in the environment or visit a department with clinical alarms to assess the impact of alarms.

These exercises can be accomplished in a discussion occurring in the physical classroom, in an online synchronous classroom, or in a facilitator-prompted course-platform-based discussion board.

STUDENT EVALUATION

Facilitators should evaluate the following:

12.1 Was the student able to articulate the definition and implications of alarm fatigue?
12.2 Was the student able to apply knowledge gained from reading to identify sources and potential failure modes of clinical alarms?

CHAPTER 13

INNOVATIVE TECHNOLOGY, STANDARDIZATION, AND THE IMPACT ON HIGH RELIABILITY

In this chapter, students will learn how new and innovative technology, automation, standardization, and forcing functions are effective approaches to making a process highly reliable. Students will also learn that successful integration of technologies requires a systematic approach, an understanding of the learning health system, and a commitment to patient safety as a foundational value to achieve highly reliable performance.

Learning Objective

Examine how technology can be used to effectively hardwire processes and improve results.

Learning Activity 13.1: Apply Knowledge of Effective Interventions for High Reliability to Analyze Technological Advances in Your Practice

Learning Activity Objectives

13.1 Discuss technology and its impact on high reliability in your environment (*understanding*).

13.2 Analyze current safety interventions from your experience and place them in the Institute for Safe Medication Practices (ISMP) hierarchy of interventions (*analyzing*).

13.3 Discuss the significance of workarounds, including why workarounds occur and how to mitigate them (*understanding*).

Preparation

Prior to completion of the learning activity, students should:

- Read Chapter 13.
- Read "Nurse Workarounds in the Electronic Health Record: An Integrative Review" at https://doi.org/10.1093/jamia/ocaa050.
- Read "Human Factors Engineering" at https://psnet.ahrq.gov/primer/human-factors-engineering.
- Read "Education as a Low-Value Improvement Intervention: Often Necessary but Rarely Sufficient" at https://doi.org/10.1136/bmjqs-2019-010411.

Instructions

13.1 Assess your work environment. List examples of how technology is used and what impact it has on patient safety and high reliability. Consider the following in the discussion:

- How does the technology improve workflow?
- How does the technology improve communication?
- How does the technology improve patient safety?
- Do end users see the value of the technology?
- Are there any unexpected consequences that were found after implementation?

13.2 Use the ISMP hierarchy and list examples of each level of the hierarchy in relation to your practice and prevention of high-risk events. Also, list the pros and cons and safety effectiveness of each level (see Table 13.1).

Answer Example:

TABLE 13.1 APPLYING THE ISMP HIERARCHY FOR PREVENTION OF HIGH-RISK EVENTS

	Example in Practice	Pros	Cons	How Does This Improve Individual Safety?	How Does This Improve System Safety?	Will This Prevent the Error From Recurring?
Education and information	Staff frequently miss turning bed alarms back on, and patients are falling. Staff are educated in a staff meeting to remember to turn on the bed alarm when leaving a room.	The staff at the meeting hear the request and may remember to be more careful.	Absent or temporary staff do not hear the message.	Weak effect	Weak effect	Not likely
Rules and policies	A policy is created that states that staff "will turn the bed alarm on" prior to leaving a room.	The policy will be followed if it is disseminated and visible to staff	Staff may not be able to find policy, do not know of policy, and do not comply.	Stronger than education but only if the policy is visible.	Can drive accountability, but a policy alone does not produce outcomes.	Only for staff aware of the policy
Checklists and double-check systems	Room exit checklist hung on the inside of the door that states "Did you turn the bed alarm on?"	A reminder in real time can be helpful.	Signs and checklists can be ignored.	Moderate effect	Moderate effect	Visual cues to double check can be helpful in real time, and a visible reminder may prevent this error.
Standardization and protocols	Documentation is added on an hourly basis to document that the bed alarm is on.	This standardization by documenting serves as a reminder and a priority.	Unless this is mandatory documentation, it could be ignored.	Moderate effect	Moderate effect	This may reinforce the priority for all staff who are documenting care for the patient.
Automation and computerization	A trigger is added to the bed alarm to sound an alarm when it is turned off.	This serves as an auditory reminder to staff to reset the bed alarm.	The alarm could be silenced and serve as another type of alarm fatigue.	Moderate effect	Moderate effect	This auditory reminder could be very effective.

	Example in Practice	Pros	Cons	How Does This Improve Individual Safety?	How Does This Improve System Safety?	Will This Prevent the Error From Recurring?
Forcing functions and constraints	A function is added to the bed alarm that sends a signal to the primary nurse or aide when an activated alarm is off.	Missed bed alarms will be noticed and corrected quickly.	The staff who receive the message would need to promptly respond.	High effect	High effect	Highly likely if response time is effective.

13.3 The goal of high reliability strategies is to make it easier to do the right thing and harder to do the wrong thing. Workarounds are commonly created because it is difficult to do the right thing. Discuss workarounds to various practices, why they were created, and how to mitigate them. See the example in Table 13.2.

Answer Example:

TABLE 13.2 ANALYSIS OF WORKAROUNDS

Safety Technology	Workaround	Why Does It Exist?	How Can It Be Fixed?
Example: Bedside scanning of medications	Lack of scanning at bedside	Scanner doesn't reach the bedside and is attached to the computer	Wireless scanner

LEARNING ACTIVITY IMPLEMENTATION

Students will benefit the most from these exercises by doing them individually rather than in a group. The exercises are best completed with students applying the knowledge learned to their own experience.

For Exercise 13.1, students should assess their work environment. They should list examples of how technology is used and how it affects patient safety and high reliability. If any students do not have a practice environment, encourage them to interview a clinician in their field of interest to obtain the work environment examples.

For Exercise 13.2, students use the ISMP hierarchy and table template. Students should list examples of each level of the hierarchy in relation to their practice and prevention of high-risk events. Facilitators should remind students to include a list of the pros and cons and safety effectiveness of each level.

For Exercise 13.3, facilitators should focus students on workarounds. They should encourage students to discuss workarounds to various practices in their practice environment. Facilitators should coach students to include why workarounds are created and how workarounds can be learning opportunities for improvement.

These exercises can be accomplished in a discussion occurring in the physical classroom, in an online synchronous classroom, or in an facilitator-prompted course-platform-based discussion board. A short, graded paper with references discussing technology, pros and cons, effect on patient safety, and inherent workarounds is an option.

STUDENT EVALUATION

Facilitators should evaluate the following:

13.1 Was the student able to evaluate current technology in their practice and the impact (or not) on safety and reliability?

13.2 Was the student able to articulate how the ISMP hierarchy of interventions relates to high reliability?

13.3 Was the student able to articulate the meaning of workarounds and why they are created?

CHAPTER 14

TIERED SAFETY HUDDLES

In this chapter, students will learn about the concept of a tiered safety huddle as a strategy to maintain an awareness of operational conditions in an HRO. Students will also learn about how tiered safety huddles used to ensure problems from the front line of care are escalated to higher levels within the organization for awareness, system accountability, and resolution of the problem.

Learning Objective

Examine the tiered safety huddle as a vehicle to increase organization and system situational awareness.

Learning Activity 14.1: Describe the Value of the Tiered Huddle in Healthcare as an Effective Tool to Promote High Reliability in a Complex Organization

Learning Activity Objectives

14.1 Describe the purpose and the value of a tiered huddle to patient safety and quality (*understanding*).

14.2 Appraise the tiered huddle intervention as an effective tool within a complex environment (*analyzing*).

Preparation

Prior to completion of the learning activity, students should:

- Read Chapter 14.
- Read "Tiered Safety Huddles Target Zero Harm" at https://www.todayshospitalist.com/tiered-safety-huddles-target-zero-harm/.
- Read "Creating a Process for the Implementation of Tiered Huddles in a Veterans Affairs Medical Center" at https://doi.org/10.1093/milmed/usac073.

Instructions

14.1 Assess your current work environment or interview a clinician in a healthcare work environment using the following questions (see Table 14.1).

TABLE 14.1 PROBLEM AND ERROR IDENTIFICATION FOR FRONTLINE CARE PROVIDERS

Interview Questions	Response Notes
How are problems surfaced by those at the front line of care?	
How often do those from the front line bring up issues?	
Is there a formal mechanism to ensure these issues are recorded and escalated to those who can resolve the problems?	
Are your senior leaders aware of the daily challenges at the front line of care?	
Are senior leaders made aware of these challenges on a daily basis?	
What is the senior leader's role and response to resolve daily challenges?	
How does the resolution make it back to the front line?	

Interview Questions	Response Notes
How do issues that involve the "system"—such as complex processes and procedures, equipment issues, and contract issues—get resolved?	
How are problems surfaced by those at the front line of care?	
How often do those from the front line bring up issues?	

14.2 Search the literature to consider healthcare as a complex system. Discuss the following:

- Define a complex system.
- List characteristics of healthcare systems that contribute to complexity.
- Discuss how a tiered huddle contributes to all principles of high reliability.
- How does a tiered huddle provide a mechanism to handle aspects of complexity?

LEARNING ACTIVITY IMPLEMENTATION

Students will benefit most from these exercises when they do them individually rather than in a group.

Exercise 14.1 can be completed as a structured classroom discussion or as an online discussion. The objective is to assess how frontline issues are escalated or not escalated within the student's organization to explain the value of the tiered huddle.

Exercise 14.2 can be completed as a graded paper with references or as an online posting. The purpose is to understand complexity in healthcare, connect high reliability principles, and connect the tiered huddle as an effective intervention in a complex environment.

These exercises can be accomplished in a discussion occurring in the physical classroom, in an online synchronous classroom, or in a facilitator-prompted course-platform-based discussion board. A short, graded paper with references is an option.

STUDENT EVALUATION

Facilitators should evaluate the following:

14.1 Was the student able to describe the characteristic and the purpose of the tiered huddle?

14.2 Was the student able to articulate the value of the tiered huddle as a vehicle to promote high reliability principles within a complex healthcare environment?

PART V

HRO CONCEPTS AND APPLICATION TO PRACTICE: DEFERENCE TO EXPERTISE

Learning Objective

Recommend quality and safety activities based on high reliability principles (*evaluating*).

Contents

Chapter 15 The Current Need for Interprofessional Collaborative Care and Teamwork 77

Chapter 16 Meaningful Patient Engagement: Best Practice for High Reliability 81

Chapter 17 Pediatric Patient Safety: Utilizing Safety Coaching as a Strategy Toward Zero Harm 84

CHAPTER 15

THE CURRENT NEED FOR INTERPROFESSIONAL COLLABORATIVE CARE AND TEAMWORK

In this chapter, students will learn about how an increased focus on quality, safety, and efficiency in healthcare has placed greater attention on understanding the complexity of healthcare teams. Students will also learn about interprofessional collaboration and teamwork in the context of HROs.

Learning Objective

Illustrate interprofessional collaboration and teamwork in the context of HROs.

Learning Activity 15.1: Describe and Explain an Interprofessional Team in the Context of HROs

Learning Activity Objectives

15.1 Describe interprofessional collaboration in the context of HROs (*understanding*).

15.2 Explain teamwork in the context of HROs (*applying*).

Preparation

Prior to completion of the learning activity, students should:

- Read Chapter 15.
- Read "Teamwork in Healthcare: Key Discoveries Enabling Safer, High-Quality Care" at https://doi.org/10.1037/amp0000298.
- Read "Creating a Culture of Teamwork Through the Use of the TeamSTEPPS Framework: A Review of the Literature and Considerations for Nurse Practitioners" at https://doi.org/10.12806/V21/I1/R11.
- Consider characteristics of effective interprofessional teams.
- Consider evidence-based tools that support teams in assessing the current state to best identify short-term goals for improving team function.

Instructions

15.1 Describe the characteristics of an interprofessional collaborative team in your organization. Include an assessment of the strength and weaknesses of the team using one evidence-based tool (see Table 15.1).

Answer Example:

TABLE 15.1 INTERPROFESSIONAL COLLABORATIVE TEAM ASSESSMENT

Interprofessional Team Name: CAUTI Prevention Team	
Team Characteristics	Description
Team leadership	Clear, common purpose
	Clear role definition for each member
	Work assigned thoughtfully to content expert
	Members involved in decision-making
Trust	Team members able to voice disagreements without fear of retaliation
	Conflict effectively managed
Backup behavior	Team decision-making process tries to make efficacious recommendations for all patients

CHAPTER 15 THE CURRENT NEED FOR INTERPROFESSIONAL COLLABORATIVE CARE AND TEAMWORK

Team Assessment Using the Evidence-Based Assessment Tool: Team Decision-Making Questionnaire (TDMQ)	
Strengths	*Weaknesses*
Conflict effectively managed	Clinical staff's perception of decision-making
Trust	Shared mental model

15.2 Based on your assessment, make recommendations on how to strengthen the performance of the interprofessional collaborative team in the context of an HRO. Include one team training strategy and rationale for use (see Table 15.2).

Answer Example:

TABLE 15.2 RECOMMENDATIONS FOR INTERPROFESSIONAL COLLABORATIVE TEAM IMPROVEMENT

Weakness	Recommendation for Improvement (include team training strategy with rationale)	High Reliability Context (link to high reliability principles)
Example: Clinical staff's perception of decision-making	TeamSTEPPS training to facilitate development of a shared mental model and development of continuous team communication to improve staff's perception of decision-making	Commitment to resilience

LEARNING ACTIVITY IMPLEMENTATION

Students will benefit most from these learning activities when an interprofessional team at the student organization is used for the learning activities. Optimally, the student should be a member of the interprofessional team.

For Exercise 15.1, students assess strengths and weaknesses of an interprofessional team using one of the evidence-based tools presented in the chapter. Students must include characteristics of effective teams in the discussion.

For Exercise 15.2, students make recommendations to strengthen the interprofessional team based on the assessment completed in Learning Activity 15.1. Recommendations must include one team training strategy along with rationale for use. In addition, students should link team characteristics to high reliability in the discussion.

These exercises can be accomplished in a discussion occurring in the physical classroom, in an online synchronous classroom, or in a facilitator-prompted course-platform-based discussion board. Also, facilitators may consider this exercise as a graded paper or student presentation to the class.

STUDENT EVALUATION

Facilitators should evaluate the following:

15.1 Was the student able to identify and describe the characteristics of an interprofessional team? Was assessment of team strengths and weaknesses completed using an evidence-based tool?

15.2 Was the student able to make recommendations to improve team performance that included one team training strategy? Was the student able to link effective team characteristics and high reliability principles?

CHAPTER 16

MEANINGFUL PATIENT ENGAGEMENT: BEST PRACTICE FOR HIGH RELIABILITY

In this chapter, students will learn about healthcare organizations' focus on meaningful patient engagement in the context of high reliability efforts such as quality and safety improvement. Students will also learn about methods commonly used to partner with patients and families, as well as practical strategies to approximate and sustain partnerships.

Learning Objective

Explore how partnership and collaboration with patients contributes to the achievement of a consistent, highly reliable patient experience.

Learning Activity 16.1: Explain Meaningful Patient and Family Engagement in the Context of High Reliability for Patient Safety and Quality

Learning Activity Objectives

16.1 Identify co-producing opportunities for patient and family engagement in an organization (*applying*).

16.2 Analyze various patient and family engagement methodological approaches to create meaningful partnerships in safety and quality improvement (*analyzing*).

Preparation

Prior to completion of the learning activity, students should:

- Read Chapter 16.
- Read "Guide to Patient and Family Engagement in Hospital Quality and Safety" at https://www.ahrq.gov/patient-safety/patients-families/engagingfamilies/index.html.

Instructions

16.1 Describe how to empower patients and families across patient and family engagement opportunities (see Table 16.1).

Answer Example:

TABLE 16.1 EXAMPLE: ENGAGING AND EMPOWERING PATIENTS AND FAMILIES

Level of Engagement	Ways to Engage and Empower Patients and Families	Example(s)	Facilitator(s)	Barrier(s)
Process of care	Educate to improve the self-management of their conditions and empower them for shared decision-making Invest in their knowledge, skills, and attitudes related to their own patient safety	Care decisions, planning goals, bedside shift report, teach-back	Tools and workflows for patients and families to improve condition, self-care management, and safety	Patients too sick to be involved in self-care management Partnership with family members to improve condition, self-management, and safety
Practice, organizational, community, and policy	Learn from and with patients and care partners who experience unsafe care to improve understanding of the nature of harm and foster the development of more effective solutions	Patient and family advisor members are standing members of safety and quality improvement projects	Patients and healthcare professionals recognize the value of quality and safety projects	Inconveniences due to a lack of time and difficulty recruiting patient and family advisors

16.2 In a 500-word essay, discuss how to create meaningful patient and family partnerships in a safety or quality initiative. Identify a safety or quality improvement opportunity from the literature or at your organization and discuss how you could codesign the project to create meaningful patient and family partnerships. Include the following in your discussion:

- Collaborate with senior leaders
- Build trusting relationships and instill confidence
- Recruit and retain participants
- Empower the voice of patients and families
- Power dynamics
- Diverse perspectives
- Facilitators and barriers

LEARNING ACTIVITY IMPLEMENTATION

Students will benefit the most from these learning activities when they do them in a group of four or five students.

For Exercise 16.1, students should be able to describe how to empower patients and families across patient and family engagement opportunities. Students should be able to generate a table that links level of engagement with ways to engage patients and families with examples, as well as facilitators and barriers.

For Exercise 16.2, students identify a safety or quality improvement opportunity and discuss how they could codesign a project to create meaningful patient and family partnerships. Facilitators should facilitate student discussion to connect project conceptualization to creating meaningful partnerships.

These exercises can be accomplished in a discussion occurring in the physical classroom, in an online synchronous classroom, or in a facilitator-prompted course-platform-based discussion board. These exercises could also be a graded paper.

STUDENT EVALUATION

Facilitators should evaluate the following:

16.1 Was the student able to describe how to empower patients and families across patient and family engagement opportunities?

16.2 Was the student able to identify a safety or quality improvement opportunity and discuss how they could codesign a project to create meaningful patient and family partnerships?

CHAPTER 17

PEDIATRIC PATIENT SAFETY: UTILIZING SAFETY COACHING AS A STRATEGY TOWARD ZERO HARM

In this chapter, students will learn about the difficulty of sustaining successful culture change. Students will also learn that taking culture change to the front line through peer safety coaches is an effective intervention to reinforce and sustain zero harm culture.

Learning Objective

Describe implementation of a safety coach program that improved and created a platform for sustainability of HRO principles within a pediatric environment.

Learning Activity 17.1: Examine the Role of Safety Coaches as a Vehicle for Successful Change Management and Sustainability of HRO Principles

Learning Activity Objectives

17.1 Describe factors that influence change (*remembering*).

17.2 Describe the role of the patient safety coach and why it is needed for high reliability and sustained culture change (*remembering*).

17.3 Examine challenges with peer coaching and suggest solutions (*applying*).

Preparation

Prior to completion of the learning activity, students should do:

- Read Chapter 17.
- Read "How Peer Coaching Can Make Work Less Lonely" at https://hbr.org/2018/10/how-peer-coaching-can-make-work-less-lonely.
- Watch the video *Peer to Peer Coaching* at https://www.ahrq.gov/hai/cusp/videos/07d-peer-2-peer-coach/index.html.
- Read "Leading Change: Why Transformation Efforts Fail" at https://hbr.org/1995/03/leading-change-why-transformation-efforts-fail-2.

Instructions

17.1 Describe a recent initiative that succeeded or failed within your organization. Correlate the success or failure to characteristics within a change model.

- What was the initiative?
- Who led the initiative?
- How was the initiative received at the front line?
- What tactics were used to spread the initiative and sustain the progress? Was a change model used? Which one?
- Did the tactics succeed? Why?
- Review the Kotter (1995) article. What failure factors from the article were evident in a failure or mitigated in a success? What could have been done differently?

17.2 Examine the role of the safety coach and how safety coaches can create sustainability of a zero-harm initiative.

- Find and discuss a definition of a healthcare patient safety coach.
- What are the challenges with giving feedback to peers?

- Which is more successful: positive or negative feedback?
- What kind of training do safety coaches need?
- How can the role be supported to sustain gains in patient safety and quality?
- Describe the benefits to a safety coach program within an organization to achieve a culture change to high reliability. How is coaching from a peer different from coaching from a supervisor?

17.3 Practice safety coaching using an example from Table 17.1 or your own example to reinforce a desired safety behavior.

Answer Example:

TABLE 17.1 PRACTICING SAFETY COACHING

	What Did You Observe?	What Is the Expectation?	How Would You Coach?
Hand hygiene: Staff member does not practice hand hygiene.	Example: Staff member does not practice hand hygiene when entering a room.	Hand hygiene is expected when entering a room.	"Observations on your hand hygiene are always excellent, and I know that it is important to you. I noticed that this morning you didn't perform hand hygiene prior to going into Mr. Jones's room. Was there something else going on that was a distraction?"
Preventions of falls: Staff member leaves the room and does not set the bed alarm.	Example: You are doing rounds and find a bed alarm not set. The family member says that the nurse got called out of the room emergently after getting the patient back in bed.	Bed alarm is set.	"I was rounding and noticed that the bed alarm on Mr. Jones was not set. You always ensure that your high-risk fall patients are safe. I know you got called out of the room quickly. Is there a way that we could design a process to ensure that when someone gets called out of a high-risk room, another staff member can go in and check to see if all safety measures are in place?"
Protecting confidentiality: You hear staff members talking about a patient in the elevator.			
Effective communication: You witness a peer using a repeat-back to clarify an order.			
Asking questions: You hear a peer clarifying an unclear order.			

LEARNING ACTIVITY IMPLEMENTATION

Students will benefit most from these learning activities when they do them individually rather than in a group.

For Exercise 17.1, students should discuss principles of successful changes models. Facilitators should guide students to apply a change model to an organization initiative and analyze the outcome of the initiative within the context of the selected change model.

For Exercise 17.2, students focus on the role of the safety coach. Students should articulate the value of a safety coach program for sustainability. Facilitators should guide students to include practical challenges when providing peer-to-peer feedback.

For Exercise 17.3, students practice peer coaching through examples. Facilitators should guide students to reflect on how it feels to practice peer coaching. This is an independent activity. However, student examples can be practiced in small groups.

These exercises can be accomplished in a discussion occurring in the physical classroom, in an online synchronous classroom, or in a facilitator-prompted course-platform-based discussion board. Small groups may be conducive to practicing peer coaching.

STUDENT EVALUATION

Facilitators should evaluate the following:

17.1 Was the student able to understand and explain how successful change occurs and relate these factors to a previous initiative?

17.2 Was the student able to articulate how a safety coach program can embed culture change and sustain an HRO initiative?

17.3 Was the student able to discuss methods to provide peer-to-peer safety coaching and address challenges?

PART VI

HRO CONCEPTS AND APPLICATION TO PRACTICE: COMMITMENT TO RESILIENCE

Learning Objective

Recommend quality and safety activities based on high reliability principles (*evaluating*).

Contents

Chapter 18　Designing Resilience Into the Work Environment................89

Chapter 19　Building High Reliability Through Simulation.....................93

Chapter 20　Building Resilience Through Team Training: Rapid Response and In-Hospital Cardiac Arrests Events.............96

Chapter 21　Sustaining a Culture of Safety...100

CHAPTER 18

DESIGNING RESILIENCE INTO THE WORK ENVIRONMENT

In this chapter, students will learn about a social-ecological perspective of resilience. Students will also learn to relate this perspective to high reliability, design a resilient work environment, and associate individual and work environment resilience with clinician well-being.

Learning Objective

Discover a social-ecological perspective of resilience to support clinician well-being.

Learning Activity 18.1: Apply a Social-Ecological Perspective of Resilience to Support Clinician Well-Being in the Work Environment

Learning Activity Objectives

18.1 Describe resilience and how it relates to high reliability (*understanding*).

18.2 Discuss opportunities for designing a resilient work environment (*understanding*).

18.3 Associate individual and work environment resilience with clinician well-being (*understanding*).

Preparation

Prior to completion of the learning activity, students should do:

- Read Chapter 18.
- Read "Taking Action Against Clinician Burnout: A Systems Approach to Professional Well-Being" at https://doi.org/10.17226/25521.

Instructions

18.1 Describe resilience in your organization in the context of high reliability.

18.2 Discuss three strategies to design a more resilient work environment in your organization. Include tactics to facilitate clinician well-being (see Table 18.1).

Answer Example:

TABLE 18.1 EXAMPLE OF STRATEGIES TO DESIGN A RESILIENT WORK ENVIRONMENT

Work Environment Resilience Strategy	Tactics to Facilitate Clinician Well-Being
Leadership	Listens
	Practices stewardship to others
	Shows empathy
Culture	Respect
	Professionalism
Community	Providing and receiving social support
	Healing at the center of healthcare

18.3 Give three examples of how individual and work environment resilience affect clinician well-being within a social-ecological perspective of resilience (see Table 18.2).

Answer Example:

TABLE 18.2 EFFECTS OF INDIVIDUAL AND WORK ENVIRONMENT RESILIENCE

Social-Ecological Perspective	Individual Resilience	Workplace Environment Resilience	Clinician Well-Being Influence
Individual	Maintaining a healthy diet	Healthy foods offered in cafeteria at reasonable price	Staying healthy
Team resilience	Practicing good stress-management routines	Being alert to overload	Achieving work-life balance
Organization resilience	Supporting good stress management	Ability of clinical unit to accept a sudden influx of patients	Maintaining safety and quality
Society/external environment	Professional factors	Organization shares a common leadership approach to professional policy	Mitigating burnout

LEARNING ACTIVITY IMPLEMENTATION

Students will benefit most from these learning activities when they do them individually rather than in a group.

For Exercise 18.1, students describe resilience in the context of high reliability in their organization. Students must link the concepts of resilience and high reliability.

For Exercise 18.2, students discuss three strategies that could be employed at their organization to design a more resilient work environment. Exercise 18.2 builds on the description of resilience from Learning Activity 18.1. Facilitators should coach discussion to include association of work environment resilience strategies and tactics that could facilitate clinician well-being.

For Exercise 18.3, students provide examples of individual and work environment resilience and discuss how their examples influence clinician well-being. Facilitators should facilitate discussion framed in the social-ecological perspective explained in the chapter narrative and depicted in Figure 18.1 of the textbook.

These exercises can be accomplished in a discussion occurring in the physical classroom, in an online synchronous classroom, or in a facilitator-prompted course-platform-based discussion board. Also, facilitators may consider these exercises as a graded paper or student presentation to the class.

STUDENT EVALUATION

Facilitators should evaluate the following:

18.1 Was the student able to describe resilience in the context of high reliability?

18.2 Was the student able to discuss and associate work environment resiliency strategies with tactics that facilitate clinician well-being?

18.3 Was the student able to provide examples of how individual and work environment resilience affect well-being within the social-ecological framework?

CHAPTER 19

BUILDING HIGH RELIABILITY THROUGH SIMULATION

In this chapter, students will learn about healthcare simulation and blend simulation with the concepts of high reliability to create a view of simulation that improves the safety of high-risk processes. Students will also learn about the benefits of employing simulation as an advanced quality improvement and patient safety tool.

Learning Objective

Describe the emergence of simulation in hospitals, schools, and other healthcare organizations as an advanced quality-improvement and patient-safety tool.

Learning Activity 19.1: Explore Opportunities to Use Simulation to Improve Safety and Reliability of Risk-Prone Processes

Learning Activity Objectives

19.1 Compare and contrast traditional simulation and simulation designed for high reliability (*analyzing*).

19.2 Apply simulation to a high-risk process to improve the safety of the process (*applying*).

Preparation

Prior to completion of the learning activity, students should:

- Read Chapter 19.
- Read "Using Clinical Simulation to Study How to Improve Quality and Safety in Healthcare" at https://doi.org/10.1136/bmjstel-2018-000370.
- Find one peer-reviewed research article that applies simulation to a clinical safety or quality problem.

Instructions

19.1 In a 500-word essay, describe the difference between traditional simulation, such as experience for learning competencies, and simulation to improve safety of a high-risk process.

- List some high-risk processes from your experience that might benefit from a simulation exercise.
- How have these processes been practiced or simulated in your organization?
- Were the practice sessions realistic?
- Did the practice identify areas for improvement in teamwork, communication, or critical thinking?
- Did the practice identify potential failures that might occur in the process?
- Did participants in the practice session feel psychologically safe to speak up?
- Did debriefing occur after the practice session?
- Pick one of the high-risk processes that you currently practice or drill in your facility. Redesign the practice or drill to create a simulation that identifies safety issues within the process and increases the safety of the process.
- Describe how simulation could be combined with an FMEA to identify failure modes.

19.2 Present your research article to fellow students.

- What was the practice problem that the simulation addressed?
- Describe the method used for simulation.
- What were the objectives and outcomes of the simulation?
- Identify a high reliability principle that the simulation addressed or could have addressed.

LEARNING ACTIVITY IMPLEMENTATION

Students will benefit most from these learning activities when they do them individually rather than in a group.

For Exercise 19.1, students explore the world of simulation and how it can be used to effectively increase safety and improve quality. Facilitators guide students to compare traditional simulation that simply reflects practice and simulation designed to identify failures and encourage teamwork and resilience.

For Exercise 19.2, students present peer-reviewed research articles that apply simulation to a clinical safety or quality problem either in-person or synchronously to classmates. Facilitators should guide the discussion to more fully explore simulation as a specialty practice.

These exercises can be accomplished in a discussion occurring in the physical classroom, in an online synchronous classroom, or in a facilitator-prompted course-platform-based discussion board. Also, facilitators may consider these exercises as a graded paper or a student presentation to the class.

STUDENT EVALUATION

Facilitators should evaluate the following:

19.1 Was the student able to describe simulation for competency and simulation for high reliability?

19.2 Was the student able to identify opportunities for improved simulation of a high-risk process within the practice?

CHAPTER 20

BUILDING RESILIENCE THROUGH TEAM TRAINING: RAPID RESPONSE AND IN-HOSPITAL CARDIAC ARREST EVENTS

In this chapter, students will assess and evaluate the role resilience plays through team training events. Students will practice with an in-depth example of a healthcare emergency where multiple team members manage the emergency.

Learning Objective

Explain and evaluate how the high reliability principle of resilience improves team response to a cardiac event.

Learning Activity 20.1: Evaluate Rapid Response and In-Hospital Cardiac Arrest Event Team Performance

Learning Activity Objectives

20.1 Evaluate rapid response and in-hospital cardiac arrest event team performance (*evaluating*).

20.2 Explain team resilience gap analysis (*analyzing*).

Preparation

Prior to completion of the learning activity, students should:

- Read Chapter 20.
- Read "Empowering Nurses to Activate the Rapid Response Team" at https://www.nursingcenter.com/journalarticle?Article_ID=5563265&Journal_ID=54016&Issue_ID=5563146.

Instructions

20.1 Prepare an in-hospital cardiac arrest event team debrief using the post-code pause structured format (see Figure 20.1). Include team resilience gap analysis in your discussion.

Date:_____ Age of Patient_____ Type of Alert:_____

**Names of all staff members involved in post resuscitation pause

_____   _____

_____   _____   _____

**After the Event, everyone pauses for 10 seconds of silence to either remember the life of the person or celebrate the success of the Code Blue

What did the team do well?

What intervention(s) do you wish had or had not been offered?

How is your satisfaction with the equipment and medications available?

Where can we grow and improve?

How did we support the family (if they are present)?

How are you doing after the code?

What do you need to be able to be successful for returning to work right now?

Additional comments or concerns:

Figure 20.1 Post-code pause form.

20.2 Prepare a rapid response event team debrief using the "What's Right?" structured format. Include team resilience gap analysis in your discussion (see Table 20.1). The team leader will ask:

- Identify two things that went well in this RRT.
- Identify anything we can do to improve our RRT.

Each team member will be encouraged to share thoughts and new ideas.

TABLE 20.1 RESILIENCE QUALITIES TO CONSIDER DURING GAP ANALYSIS

Indicator	Present	Absent	Follow-Up	Outcome Date
Are red-flag events or near misses reported?				
Is reporting of red-flag events rewarded?				
Is reporting of red-flag events punished?				
Have suggestions for workflow come from the workforce level?				
Do team meetings allow time for open discussion of everyday processes?				
Is the workflow regularly observed and evaluated by others?				
Does this process allow variation, or is variation open to safety issues?				
Have there been action-based mock drills?				
Are preprocess briefings used regularly?				
Are post-event debriefings used regularly?				
Is crew resource management training used with supervisors, and are the results monitored by leadership?				
Are stressful events (with or without outcome errors) reviewed?				
Are predictable workforce stressors identified and mitigated?				
After error mitigation, is the goal to return to steady state?				
Are the values of safety supported on every level of the workforce?				
Is data about safety, productivity, or processes well known and understood at all levels of the workforce?				

LEARNING ACTIVITY IMPLEMENTATION

Students will benefit most from these learning activities when they do them in a group rather than individually.

For Exercise 20.1, the facilitator should provide a video simulation of a mock in-hospital cardiac arrest event for students to view. Divide or assign students to groups to view the video simulation, and then have each group of students prepare a debrief using the post-code pause structured format. Students should be prepared to present their observations and discuss opportunities to improve in-hospital cardiac arrest team performance, including team resilience gap analysis.

For Exercise 20.1, the facilitator should provide a video simulation of a rapid response event for students to view. Divide or assign students to groups to view the video simulation, and then have each group of students prepare a debrief using the debriefing tool "What's Right?" structured format. Students should be prepared to present their observations and discuss opportunities to help the simulation team define their strengths and areas for growth, including team resilience gap analysis.

These exercises can be accomplished in a discussion occurring in the physical classroom, in an online synchronous classroom, or in an facilitator-prompted course-platform-based discussion board.

STUDENT EVALUATION

Facilitators should evaluate the following:

20.1 Was the student able to prepare an in-hospital cardiac arrest event team debrief using the post-code pause structured format reflective of the event in the simulation video? Did the student include resilience strategies in the discussion?

20.2 Was the student able to prepare a rapid response event team debrief using the "What's Right?" structured format reflective of the event in the simulation video? Did the student include resilience strategies in the discussion?

CHAPTER 21

SUSTAINING A CULTURE OF SAFETY

In this chapter, students will learn how resilient organizations can sustain a culture of safety by creating an organizational culture of personal and professional accountability.

Learning Objective

Explore a framework for change with strategies to sustain and maintain the gains within a culture of safety.

Learning Activity 21.1: Focus on Sustaining a Culture of Safety in a Resilient Organization

Learning Activity Objectives

21.1 Discuss organizational vulnerabilities, related performance, and adherence to regulations and policies across the care continuum as a rationale for sustaining a culture of safety (*understanding*).

21.2 Apply a framework for change to sustain and maintain a culture of safety (*applying*).

21.3 Explain strategies to maintain the gains within a culture of safety in a resilient organization (*analyzing*).

Preparation

Prior to completion of the learning activity, students should:

- Read Chapter 21.
- Read *It Starts With One: Changing Individuals Changes Organizations* (3rd ed.), by J. S. Black.

Instructions

21.1 Discuss steps in developing culture change to support individual professional accountability and healthcare system performance.

21.2 Apply an evidence-based change model of your choice to a problem at your organization. Include barriers to change and mitigation strategies (see Table 21.1).

Answer Example:

TABLE 21.1 CHANGE MODEL APPLICATION

Change Model	Barriers to Change	Barrier Mitigation Strategies
Failure to see → What do we see?	Past successful mental maps "This is the way we do it here"	Clinical audit and feedback Peer review
Failure to move → How do we move?	New "right" thing not clearly identified Fear of appearing incompetent	Clear target identified Tools to help navigate to clear target—process improvement cycles
Failure to finish → How do we finish?	Fatigue—not going far enough or fast enough for change to succeed Majority do not adopt change	Champions to reinforce and encourage Majority adopt change

21.3 Name three strategies you could use after an evidence-based change to maintain and sustain gains in a culture of safety (see Table 21.2).

Answer Example:

TABLE 21.2 THREE STRATEGIES FOR GAINS IN A CULTURE OF SAFETY

Strategy	Tactics
Leadership	Formal training
	Safety is a strategic plan priority
	Active listening
Infrastructure and resource investment	Human factors engineer
	Internal governance and committee structure
Data analysis and feedback	Serious reportable events
	View multiple sources of data

LEARNING ACTIVITY IMPLEMENTATION

Students will benefit most from these learning activities when they do them in a group of four or five students.

For Exercise 21.1, students discuss the steps for developing culture change that support individual professional accountability and healthcare system performance. Students should include organizational vulnerabilities, related performance, and adherence to regulations and policies across the care continuum as a rationale for sustaining a culture of safety in their discussion.

For Exercise 21.2, students apply an evidence-based change model to a problem at their organization. The evidence-based change model for the learning activity is the student's choice. However, the model presented in Chapter 21 of the textbook is adequate for this activity. Facilitators should guide students to include barriers to change and barrier mitigation strategies in EBP model application.

For Exercise 21.3, students name three strategies to maintain and sustain a culture of safety. The students should link strategies to maintain and sustain a culture of safety and organizational resilience in their discussion.

These exercises can be accomplished in a discussion occurring in the physical classroom, in an online synchronous classroom, or in a facilitator-prompted course-platform-based discussion board. Also, facilitators may consider these exercises as a student presentation to the class.

STUDENT EVALUATION

Facilitators should evaluate the following:

21.1 Was the student able to discuss the steps to develop culture change? Did the student link individual professional accountability and health system performance to the steps of culture change?

21.2 Was the student able to select and apply an evidence-based change model to a problem at the organization? Did the student include barriers to change and mitigation strategies in the discussion?

21.3 Was the student able to name three strategies to sustain and maintain the gains following an evidence-based change?

PART VII

ASSIMILATION INTO PRACTICE ACROSS THE CONTINUUM

Learning Objective

Integrate high reliability principles into healthcare practice (*creating*).

Contents

Chapter 22   Ambulatory Care: The Frontier for High Reliability 105

Chapter 23   The Synthesis Among Magnet Recognition Program® Model Components and High Reliability Organization Principles 108

Chapter 24   Realizing High Reliability: Nurse Scientist and Bedside Scientist Collaboration 112

Chapter 25   Ensuring High Reliability in Acute Stroke Treatment 119

CHAPTER 22

AMBULATORY CARE: THE FRONTIER FOR HIGH RELIABILITY

In this chapter, students will learn about how high reliability principles can be used to address key quality and safety challenges in ambulatory care. Students will learn about the scope of ambulatory services as well as some of the unique complexities and challenges of this specialty.

Learning Objective

Discover how the principles of high reliability can mitigate quality and safety challenges in the ambulatory care setting.

Learning Activity 22.1: Integrate High Reliability Principles to Address Quality and Safety Challenges in Ambulatory Care

Learning Activity Objectives

22.1 Discuss the scope of ambulatory services and the varied ambulatory settings (*understanding*).

22.2 Explain complexities and challenges of ambulatory care (*understanding*).

22.3 Articulate how each of the principles of high reliability can be used to mitigate quality and safety challenges in the ambulatory care space (*applying*).

Preparation

Prior to completion of the learning activity, students should:

- Read Chapter 22.
- Read "The Economics of Patient Safety in Primary and Ambulatory Care: Flying Blind" at https://doi.org/10.1787/baf425ad-en.

Instructions

22.1 Choose an ambulatory care setting in your organization. Include the rationale for your choice.

22.2 Identify at least three complexities and challenges of the chosen ambulatory care setting using Table 22.1.

22.3 Continuing with Table 22.1, add high reliability principles that can mitigate complexities and challenges of the chosen ambulatory care setting.

Answer Example:

TABLE 22.1 APPLYING HIGH RELIABILITY PRINCIPLES IN AMBULATORY CARE SETTINGS

Ambulatory Care Setting: Ambulatory Infusion Center

Rationale: Outpatient administration of infusible and injectable pharmacological and biological agents. I work there.

Complexities	Unique Safety Challenges	High Reliability Solution
Diverse care team of interprofessional experts	Skill mix and delegation	Deference to expertise Clear role delineation Daily huddles
Communication gaps	Medication administration errors	Preoccupation with failure Systematic approach to reviewing errors
Care transition management	Care coordination	Sensitivity to operations Standardizing workflows and communication

LEARNING ACTIVITY IMPLEMENTATION

Students will benefit most from these learning activities when they do them individually rather than in a group.

For Exercise 22.1, students select an ambulatory care setting in their organization. Students must include a rationale for their choice.

For Exercise 22.2, students identify complexities and challenges of the ambulatory care setting from Exercise 22.1. Facilitators should facilitate discussion to include a variety of ambulatory care settings.

For Exercise 22.3, students are building on Exercise 22.1 and Exercise 22.2 by integrating high reliability principles to mitigate complexities and challenges unique to the selected ambulatory care setting. Students should be able to generate a table that links high reliability principles and strategies to mitigate complexities and challenges of the selected ambulatory care setting.

These exercises can be accomplished in a discussion occurring in the physical classroom, in an online synchronous classroom, or in a facilitator-prompted course-platform-based discussion board. Also, facilitators may consider these exercises as a graded paper or student presentation to the class.

STUDENT EVALUATION

Facilitators should evaluate the following:

22.1 Was the student able to select an ambulatory care setting in the organization? Was rationale for choice of setting included?

22.2 Was the student able to identify a minimum of three complexities and challenges of the chosen ambulatory care setting?

22.3 Was the student able to create a table integrating high reliability principles that could mitigate complexities and challenges of the selected ambulatory care setting?

CHAPTER 23

THE SYNTHESIS AMONG MAGNET RECOGNITION PROGRAM® MODEL COMPONENTS AND HIGH RELIABILITY ORGANIZATION PRINCIPLES

In this chapter, students will learn about how the Magnet® model component characteristics provide the foundation for synergistic relationships with HRO principles. Students will also learn about the synergy of Magnet components and high reliability principles.

Learning Objective

Discover how high reliability principles can be related to the components of the Magnet model.

Learning Activity 23.1: Explain the Synergistic Relationship Between the Magnet Model Components and the Principles of High Reliability

Learning Activity Objectives

23.1 Describe the Magnet Recognition Program components (*understanding*).

23.2 Discuss the synergy of high reliability principles with Magnet Recognition Program components (*understanding*).

Preparation

Prior to completion of the learning activity, students should:

- Read Chapter 23.
- Read "Magnet Model – Creating a Magnet Culture" at https://www.nursingworld.org/organizational-programs/magnet/magnet-model/.

Instructions

23.1 Discuss the five components and component characteristics of the Magnet model using Table 23.1.

   Answer Example:

TABLE 23.1 COMPONENTS AND CHARACTERISTICS OF THE MAGNET MODEL

Magnet Component	Description
1. Exemplary professional practice	Understanding of the role of nursing; autonomous practice based on competence; application of nursing role with patients, families, communities, and interprofessional teams; nurse partnerships to deliver patient-/person-centered care
2. Transformational leadership	Focuses on the quality of nursing leadership and the management style of hospital leaders. Emphasis on leaders who have vision, influence, clinical knowledge, and expertise who inspire and motivate nurses to achieve excellence and contribute to the organization's goals.
3. Structural empowerment	Organizational structures and processes that support professional practice such as organizational structure, personnel policies, professional development opportunities, and the image of nursing within the organization
4. New knowledge, innovation and improvements	Expectation is to contribute to the advancement of nursing and healthcare through research, innovation, and evidence-based practice. Emphasizes the importance of ongoing learning, new models of care, and the application of research findings to improve patient outcomes.

continues

TABLE 23.1 COMPONENTS AND CHARACTERISTICS OF THE MAGNET MODEL (CONT.)

Magnet Component	Description
5. Empirical outcomes	Integrated into the other four components, illustrating accountability for demonstrating the impact of professional nursing practice related to all components. Focus on results achieved by the organization, particularly in relation to nursing care and patient outcomes. Includes measuring and evaluating the effectiveness of structures, processes, and interventions to ensure continuous improvement.

23.2 Describe the synergy of high reliability principles and Magnet Recognition Program components and include examples of synergy using Table 23.2.

Answer Example:

TABLE 23.2 SYNERGY OF HIGH RELIABILITY AND MAGNET RECOGNITION PROGRAM

Magnet Recognition Component/ Description	Example of Magnet Component From Organization	High Reliability Principle	Description of Synergy
Transformational leadership	Vision of elimination of patient harm	Preoccupation with failure	For the preoccupation with failure to work, there needs to be a high level of trust and communication within the organization. Leadership must take time to provide the "why" and encourage two-way feedback among management and staff, and it needs to be viewed as constructive. Leaders who take the time to answer why will produce a workforce with buy-in and one that is more flexible and responsive to change.

LEARNING ACTIVITY IMPLEMENTATION

Students will benefit most from these learning activities when they do them individually rather than in a group.

For Exercise 23.1, students should be able to name each of the five components of the Magnet model. Facilitators should coach students to include description and component characteristics in their discussion.

For Exercise 23.2, students build on knowledge from Exercise 23.1. In this exercise students describe the synergy of high reliability principles and Magnet Recognition Program components by providing examples from their organization. Facilitators may need to coach students to link high reliability principles and Magnet Recognition Program components to examples in practice.

These exercises can be accomplished in a discussion occurring in the physical classroom, in an online synchronous classroom, or in a facilitator-prompted course-platform-based discussion board.

STUDENT EVALUATION

Facilitators should evaluate the following:

23.1 Was the student able to discuss the components of the Magnet model? Was the student able to discuss the characteristics of each component of the model?

23.2 Was the student able to provide practice examples describing the synergy of high reliability principles and Magnet Recognition Program components?

CHAPTER 24

REALIZING HIGH RELIABILITY: NURSE SCIENTIST AND BEDSIDE SCIENTIST COLLABORATION

In this chapter, students will learn about the collaborative relationship of bedside scientists and nurse scientists in an HRO. Students will also learn about a proposed framework to facilitate organizational quality improvement, evidence-based practice and research agendas, and infrastructure supporting the conduct of nursing research in a highly reliable organization.

Learning Objective

Explain the collaborative, synergistic relationship between nurse scientists and bedside scientists to promote a culture of safety and inquiry in an HRO.

Learning Activity 24.1: Discover the Role of the Nurse Scientist and Bedside Scientist in a High Reliability Organization

Learning Activity Objectives

24.1 Explain the role of the nurse scientist and bedside scientist in an HRO (*understanding*).

24.2 Summarize the collaborative relationship between the nurse scientist and bedside scientist in an HRO (*understanding*).

Preparation

Prior to completion of the learning activity, students should:

- Read Chapter 24.
- Read "How to Improve: Model for Improvement" at https://www.ihi.org/resources/how-improve-model-improvement.
- Read "The Role of the Nurse Scientist and Nursing Research Within a National Integrated Health Care System" at https://doi.org/10.1097/NAQ.0000000000000644.
- Read "Why Nursing Research Matters" at https://doi.org/10.1097/NNA.0000000000001005.
- Read "What Is Evidence-Based Practice in Nursing?" at https://www.nursingworld.org/content-hub/resources/workplace/evidence-based-practice-in-nursing/.

Instructions

24.1 Identify a project idea at your organization, describe the role of the nurse scientist and bedside scientist in your project, determine what type of project is best for your idea, and conduct a brief literature review on the topic (see examples in Table 24.1 and the literature review template in Table 24.2).

Answer Example:

Project Idea: Improve the medical-surgical (M/S) nursing work environment when resources are limited. Design a research study to describe the effects of implementing intermittent virtual RN support when RN personnel resources were not available to meet the agreed upon M/S unit staffing plan.

What is the role of the nurse scientist in the project?

- Guide development of a research study in collaboration with nurse leaders and clinical nursing staff
- Coach the team to develop research questions; review the literature; design the study; develop measurement tools; design a virtual nursing education program; implement the virtual nursing model study intervention; develop a statistical analysis plan; and collect, analyze, and interpret data
- Facilitate IRB approval process
- Coach the team to develop and submit a conference abstract, develop presentation for national conference, or write and submit a manuscript for publication

What is the role of the bedside scientist in the project?

- Bedside scientists discuss how to improve the nursing work environment when resources are limited
- Determine best idea to improve work environment is to ask "just in time" enterprise pool staff to meet staffing plan
- Invent, develop, and design an intermittent virtual nursing model
- Act as co-investigators at study sites
- Present study results at national conference or contribute to writing manuscript for publication

TABLE 24.1 EXAMPLES: NURSE SCIENTIST AND BEDSIDE SCIENTIST ROLES PROJECT

PROJECT TYPE:	Definition/Purpose	Rationale	Methodology
Quality improvement	Definition: Data-driven systematic approach to improve specific internal processes to meet established quality benchmarks within an organization Purpose: Improves processes to enhance quality and efficiencies	Incorporates existing knowledge into process improvement activities	Practice changes may be implemented, evaluated, and changed in succession until benchmarks are acceptable. These processes are sometimes referred to as *cycles of change*. Multiple methodologies: PDSA (Plan, Do, Study, Act), Six Sigma, Lean Six-Sigma
Evidence-based practice	Definition: A problem-solving approach in which the best available evidence, clinical expertise, and a patient's preferences or circumstances are integrated to provide optimal patient care Purpose: Improve patient care based on integration of the strongest available evidence	Translates new knowledge into clinical practice	EBP model such as Iowa, ARCC, ACE Star, Johns Hopkins, PARiHS, Stetler
Research	Definition: The systematic investigation into a phenomenon Purpose: Generation of new knowledge	Generates new knowledge for the discipline and assists in scientifically testing theories or interventions	Scientific method—quantitative, qualitative, or mixed methods

TABLE 24.2 LITERATURE REVIEW TEMPLATE

LITERATURE REVIEW				
Source (Author, Title, Year)	Purpose of Study	Method (including setting and sample)	Key Findings and Implications	Limitations of Study
Schuelke, S., Aurit, S., Connot, N., & Denney, S. (2019). Virtual nursing: the new reality in quality care. *Nursing Administration Quarterly, 43*(4), 322-328.	The purpose of this quality project was to examine the effect of the virtually integrated care team and 6 case uses on patient satisfaction, staff satisfaction, physician satisfaction, patient quality metrics, and financial metrics.	Two general medical-surgical units at different community hospitals in a large health system were utilized for the project. Site A was equipped with 20 patient rooms with virtual capabilities, which were contained on a 48-bed unit, with 24 hours per 7 days a week VN coverage. Site B was equipped with 24 patient rooms with virtual capabilities and encompassed the entire unit. Data were collected over a two-and-a-half-year period.	Patient satisfaction: 58% of patients preferred to be in a room with virtual capabilities; 17% had no preference and 25% preferred not to be in a room with virtual capabilities Staff satisfaction: The Agency for Healthcare Research and Quality survey results showed that percent positive scores improved from baseline each year at both sites. Physician satisfaction: no statically significant changes in physician satisfaction Patient quality metrics: The National Database of Nursing Quality Indicators quality metrics were monitored throughout the project, meeting, or exceeding benchmarks most quarters. Financial metrics: Site A and site B both demonstrated statistically significant decrease in labor cost per unit of service.	Not RCT Findings not generalizable

24.2 Describe the synergistic actions the bedside scientist and the nurse scientist could take to advance your project in a highly reliable organization (see Table 24.3 for examples).

Answer Example:

TABLE 24.3 BEDSIDE SCIENTIST AND NURSE SCIENTIST SYNERGIES

HRO Principles	Definition (Weick & Sutcliffe, 2015)	Nurse Scientist Actions (Kim et al., 2024)	Bedside Scientist Actions (Dunning, 2013; Stutzman et al., 2016)
Sensitivity to operations	Awareness of how processes, systems, and individual actions impact the whole organization	Bridge operational goals with organizational needs and priorities through robust research, EBP and QI agendas Conduct research on topics that align with operational or organizational needs	Bring awareness of processes and functions beyond your work group Identify problematic clinical practice issues Engage at an individual level
Preoccupation with failure	Think of ways work processes might break down	Provide immediate EBP recommendations or guidance in response to questions and requests Build capacity for EBP and nursing research by providing education related to research, EBP, and QI	Identify problematic clinical practice issues Assist in developing research questions to address clinical practice issues Evidence-based clinical nursing practice
Deference to expertise	Listen to people who have the most developed knowledge of the task at hand	Partner with professional development teams and unit-based councils to empower clinical nurse bedside scientists to use EBP and advance nursing science Build capacity for EBP and nursing research by providing education related to appraisal of the evidence, research methods, and analytics Mentor bedside scientists to apply evidence into practice and conduct research Act as a subject matter expert for EBP and research activities	Identify clinical practice questions Assist in developing research questions to address clinical practice issues Complete a Bedside Scientist Clinical Nurse Research Fellowship Program Identify a research mentor

HRO Principles	Definition (Weick & Sutcliffe, 2015)	Nurse Scientist Actions (Kim et al., 2024)	Bedside Scientist Actions (Dunning, 2013; Stutzman et al., 2016)
Reluctance to simplify	Reluctance to accept explanation of problem and dig deeper into the solution of a situation or issue	Be a subject matter expert on committees and councils Consult and serve as a leader or facilitator on research committees, unit-based practice councils, etc., to advance nursing science	Assist in developing research questions to address clinical practice issues Provide information about feasibility of implementing research methodology in clinical setting Ensure clinicians' perspectives are encompassed in study findings and recommendations
Commitment to resilience	Continuous learning and teamwork across units	Provide education related to appraisal of the evidence, research methods, and data analytics Provide education related to scholarly activities such as abstract writing, poster and podium presentation preparation and delivery, and publication Provide EBP recommendations or guidance to immediate questions or requests Build robust research, EBP, and QI teams to facilitate continuous learning and teamwork Mentor bedside scientists in scholarly activities	Become QI, EBP, and research literate Join a QI, EBP, or research team Help implement the study Assist with data collection Ensure clinicians' perspectives are encompassed in study findings and recommendations Participate in scholarly activities

LEARNING ACTIVITY IMPLEMENTATION

Students will benefit most from these learning activities when they do them either individually or in a group.

For Exercise 24.1, students should identify a project idea at their organization. Students should describe the project role of the nurse scientist and bedside scientist. Students should determine if their project idea is QI, EBP or research. Students should conduct a brief literature review on the topic. Facilitators should guide students to include three or four peer-reviewed sources of evidence on the improvement or innovation topic.

For Exercise 24.2, students build on Exercise 24.1. In this exercise students should describe the role of the nurse scientist and bedside scientist to advance their project idea within a framework of synergy grounded in the principles of high reliability. Facilitators should guide students to link high reliability to a culture of inquiry.

These exercises can be accomplished in a discussion in the physical classroom, in an online synchronous classroom, or in a facilitator-prompted course-platform-based discussion board. Facilitators may consider these exercises as a presentation to the class.

STUDENT EVALUATION

Facilitators should evaluate the following:

24.1 Was the student able to identify a project idea at their organization? Was the student able to locate three or four peer-reviewed sources of evidence from the literature on the opportunity for improvement or innovation?

24.2 Was the student able to describe how the nurse scientist and bedside scientist would collaboratively advance the project idea within a framework of synergy grounded in the principles of high reliability? Was the student able to link high reliability to a culture of inquiry?

CHAPTER 25

ENSURING HIGH RELIABILITY IN ACUTE STROKE TREATMENT

In this chapter, students will learn about how high reliability principles can be used to build a highly reliable team. Students will learn about how an acute stroke team used quality tools and change management strategies to implement a critical medication conversion.

Learning Objective

Explore the process of successful identification of failures and planning for change in large and small initiatives.

Learning Activity 25.1: Apply High Reliability Principles to Acute Stroke Treatment

Learning Activity Objectives

25.1 Show several fundamental factors that encourage or act as barriers to successful change in healthcare (*understanding*).

25.2 Apply the methods used in the chapter to a familiar example of a clinical practice change that either went well or did not go well (*applying*).

Preparation

Prior to completion of the learning activity, students should:

- Read Chapter 25.

Instructions

25.1 Identify and discuss a successful change initiative in your organization. What made it possible? Identify and discuss a change initiative in your organization that was *not* successful. What were the items that led to an unsuccessful implementation?

25.2 Identify the items in the chapter that led to a successful implementation. Discuss several of these items and how they might have improved the outcomes in the unsuccessful implementation identified in 25.1.

LEARNING ACTIVITY IMPLEMENTATION

Students will benefit the most from these learning activities when they do them individually or in a group.

For Exercise 25.1, students identify a successful and unsuccessful change initiative in their organization. Students should be able to discuss what made a change initiative successful and what made a change initiative unsuccessful. The opportunity can be from the literature if needed.

For Exercise 25.2, students review the successful implementation of a change initiative incorporating the principles of high reliability. Students should apply principles of high reliability to the unsuccessful change initiative identified in Exercise 25.1. Students should be able to explain how application of high reliability principles, change management strategies, and quality tools could improve implementation of the change initiative.

These exercises can be accomplished in a discussion occurring in the physical classroom, in an online synchronous classroom, or in a facilitator-prompted course-platform-based discussion board. Also, facilitators may consider these exercises as a graded paper or student presentation to the class.

STUDENT EVALUATION

Facilitators should evaluate the following:

25.1 Did the student identify a successful and unsuccessful change initiative in their organization?

25.2 Was the student able to apply principles of high reliability, change management strategies, and quality tools to an unsuccessful initiative that could improve implementation of the change initiative?

PART VIII

TRANSLATION INTO PRACTICE

Learning Objective

Integrate high reliability principles into healthcare practice (*creating*).

Contents

Chapter 26   High Reliability Performance During a Pandemic.............123

Chapter 27   Building a High Reliability Head and Neck Operating Room Team.......................126

Chapter 28   Decreasing Harm From Workplace Violence......................131

Chapter 29   Introduction of High Reliability to Frontline Staff: Creating a Virtual Resource Toolkit..................134

CHAPTER 26

HIGH RELIABILITY PERFORMANCE DURING A PANDEMIC

In this chapter, students will learn how infectious disease outbreaks can be anticipated. Students will learn about infectious disease outbreak interventions using the principles of high reliability and a target for zero preventable harm.

Learning Objective

Describe identification and prevention of the spread of infectious diseases.

Learning Activity 26.1: Explore High Reliability Performance During a Pandemic

Learning Activity Objectives

26.1 Explain lessons learned from the COVID-19 pandemic (*understanding*).

26.2 Apply high reliability principles in emergent infectious disease response (*applying*).

Preparation

Prior to completion of the learning activity, students should:

- Read Chapter 26.
- Read "Adapting and Creating Healing Environments: Lessons Nurses Have Learned From the COVID-19 Pandemic" at https://doi.org/10.1016/j.mnl.2021.10.013.

Instructions

26.1 Discuss the potential for the next pandemic, include what was learned from the COVID-19 experience that could be applied to future pandemics and whether we are better prepared.

26.2 Reflect on your healthcare organization's approach to the COVID-19 pandemic. Include the following in your reflection:

- How did the organization prevent panic?
- How did the organization communicate changes in the emergent environment?
- What was successful?
- What was not successful?
- Identify high reliability principles used when creating solutions in the rapidly changing context.

LEARNING ACTIVITY IMPLEMENTATION

Students will benefit the most from these learning activities when they do them individually or in a group.

For Exercise 26.1, students discuss what was learned during the COVID-19 pandemic that could be applied to future pandemics. Students should include level of preparedness for the next pandemic in the discussion.

For Exercise 26.2, students should reflect on a healthcare organization's approach to the COVID-19 pandemic. Students should include what approaches were successful and not successful in their reflection. Students should discuss how application of high reliability principles is an effective approach and give examples.

These exercises can be accomplished in a discussion occurring in the physical classroom, in an online synchronous classroom, or in a facilitator-prompted course-platform-based discussion board. Also, facilitators may consider these exercises as a graded paper or student presentation to the class.

STUDENT EVALUATION

Facilitators should evaluate the following:

26.1 Did the student's discussion of potential for the next pandemic include lessons learned from COVID-19 and preparedness for future pandemics?

26.2 Was the student able to discuss an organizational approach to the COVID-19 pandemic that includes principles of high reliability?

CHAPTER 27

BUILDING A HIGH RELIABILITY HEAD AND NECK OPERATING ROOM TEAM

In this chapter, students will learn about how high reliability principles can be used to build a highly reliable team. Students will learn about how an operating room team made the journey to becoming and continuing to be a highly reliable surgical team.

Learning Objective

Explore how to leverage high reliability principles on an interprofessional team to improve patient safety.

Learning Activity 27.1: Apply High Reliability Principles to Solve Team Quality and Safety Challenges

Learning Activity Objectives

27.1 Apply HRO characteristics to design an interprofessional team practice change that improves a quality/safety measure (*applying*).

27.2 Select an interprofessional team quality/safety improvement opportunity where application of high reliability could make a positive impact (*applying*).

27.3 Design a team project plan using the principles of high reliability to improve the interprofessional team quality/safety opportunity (*creating*).

Preparation

Prior to completion of the learning activity, students should:

- Read Chapter 27.
- Identify an interprofessional team quality/safety improvement opportunity that could be affected by team practice changes.
- Read "Nurse Leaders: Transforming Interprofessional Relationships to Bridge Healthcare Quality and Safety" at https://doi.org/10.1016/j.mnl.2021.12.003.

Instructions

27.1 Identify an interprofessional team quality/safety improvement opportunity that could be affected by team practice changes through the use of high reliability principles.

27.2 Using knowledge of high reliability principles, explain which high reliability principles are relevant in solving the problem and why (see Table 27.1).

Answer Example:

TABLE 27.1 APPLICATION OF HIGH RELIABILITY PRINCIPLES TO AN INTERPROFESSIONAL TEAM QUALITY/SAFETY IMPROVEMENT OPPORTUNITY

Quality/Safety Improvement Need	Principle 1 Preoccupation With Failure	Principle 2 Reluctance to Simplify	Principle 3 Sensitivity to Operations	Principle 4 Commitment to Resilience	Principle 5 Deference to Expertise
Reduce tissue damage during handing and management of autologous grafts during reconstructive procedures by the interprofessional operating room team.	When the surgical team constantly thinks about preventing autologous graft tissue damage, vigilance increases.	Reducing autologous graft tissue damage is a complex problem requiring intricate solutions.	Preventing autologous graft tissue is a team sport, requiring extensive interdependency of all disciplines on a surgical team.	To encourage interprofessional team commitment to reducing autologous graft tissue damage, a culture of continuous learning and support must be present.	Interprofessional team members act as subject matter experts.

27.3 Design an interprofessional team project plan using the principles of high reliability to improve the interprofessional team quality/safety opportunity. There are nine sections to complete for this activity (see Figure 27.1).

1. Describe the quality/safety project.
2. Identify the project deliverables.
3. List the baseline measures related to the project.
4. Complete the project plan charter form.
5. List steps or approaches/ideas on how you, as the team leader, would ensure integration of the high reliability principles into the solution(s).
6. Describe any risks or threats to the project.
7. Briefly describe a communication plan for the project.
8. Briefly describe a training plan for the project.
9. Briefly describe how you would evaluate the project's success.

CHAPTER 27 BUILDING A HIGH RELIABILITY HEAD AND NECK OPERATING ROOM TEAM

Potential Project Name/Title		Date	
Requested by		Charter Prepared by	

Background & Business Need: State the business problem/issue to solve or what opportunity exists to improve a business function. What is the current state? Narrative background with drivers for the project.

Project Scope Statement: Summarize the purpose and the intent of the project and describe what the customer (or you) envisions will be delivered.

Project Objectives/Deliverables: Outline the high-level objectives for the project. What will exist when the project is complete? Include the benefits of the project, including how the project will benefit the customers or stakeholders.

Boundaries: What will <u>not</u> be included in this project?

Assumptions: What assumptions were made when conceiving this project?

External Dependencies: Note any major external (to the project) dependencies the project must rely upon for success, such as specific technologies, third-party vendors, development partners, or other business relationships. Also identify any other related projects or initiatives.

Project Risks: List any known risks for the project that could impact the success of the project or should be considered when planning. Include risk of change management. Does the value of this project ultimately depend on people changing their work or behavior? Identify risks facing this project or organization if the people side of the project is poorly manned.

Key Stakeholders: List the key stakeholders for the project. Stakeholders are individuals, groups, or organizations that are actively involved in a project, are affected by its outcome, or can influence its outcome. Indicate their role or interest in the project. These stakeholders (or representatives) MAY be invited to participate in a project kickoff session but do not necessarily need to be on the project team. Whose day-to-day work will be impacted by raw processes (systems, tools, job roles, organization structure, etc.) as an outcome or deliverable of this project?

Stakeholder/Stakeholder Group	Role in Project or Impacted by This Project

Required Resources: Identify the known resources that management is willing to commit to the project at this time. Human resources includes key individuals, teams, organizations, subcontractors or vendors, and support functions. This is not the place for the detailed team staff roster for individual names. Identify critical skill sets that team members must have. Other resources could include funding, computers, other equipment, physical facilities such as buildings and rooms, hardware devices, software tools, and training. What level of change management involvement is expected for this project? (e.g., separate change management team, change management representation on the core team or individual team).

Requested Timeline/Milestones: Include end and start dates and key milestones.

Figure 27.1 Nine-step project plan template.

LEARNING ACTIVITY IMPLEMENTATION

Students will benefit the most from these learning activities when they do them in a group of four or five students.

For Exercise 27.1, students identify an interprofessional team quality/safety improvement opportunity that could be affected by team practice changes through the use of high reliability principles. The opportunity can be from their organization or from the literature.

For Exercise 27.2, students use high reliability principles to design a team practice change that improves an interprofessional team quality/safety measure by completing the table template.

For Exercise 27.3, students should design a project plan to address the interprofessional team quality/safety opportunity identified in Exercise 27.1. The nine-step project plan template is shown in Figure 27.1.

These exercises can be accomplished in a discussion occurring in the physical classroom, in an online synchronous classroom, or in a facilitator-prompted course-platform-based discussion board. Also, facilitators may consider these exercises as a graded paper or student presentation to the class.

STUDENT EVALUATION

Facilitators should evaluate the following:

27.1 Did the student select an interprofessional team quality/safety improvement opportunity that could be affected by team practice changes through the use of high reliability principles?

27.2 Was the student able to identify an interprofessional team quality/safety improvement opportunity where team practice changes can make an impact through the use of high reliability principles? Was the student able to connect how team practices connect with each high reliability principle?

27.3 Did the student design a project plan using the principles of high reliability to improve the interprofessional team quality/safety improvement opportunity?

CHAPTER 28

DECREASING HARM FROM WORKPLACE VIOLENCE

In this chapter, students will learn about workplace violence in healthcare as well as mitigation strategies. Students will also learn how application of high reliability principles and "mindful organizing" can improve workplace violence.

Learning Objective

Discuss workplace violence in healthcare experiences and successful mitigation strategies.

Learning Activity 28.1: Discuss Causes, Consequences, and Interventions to Workplace Violence in Healthcare

Learning Activity Objectives

28.1 Explain the impact of workplace violence, causes, and consequences (*understanding*).

28.2 Choose impactful interventions to decrease harm from workplace violence (*applying*).

Preparation

Prior to completion of the learning activity, students should:

- Read Chapter 28.
- Read "The Growing Burden of Workplace Violence Against Healthcare Workers: Trends in Prevalence, Risk Factors, Consequences, and Prevention – A Narrative Review" at https://doi.org/10.1016/j.eclinm.2024.102641.

Instructions

28.1 Discuss your personal experience with workplace violence as a healthcare professional. Include the following in the discussion:

- What happened?
- What was your reaction?
- What do you think provoked the violence?
- What resources were available to you to deal with it in the moment or afterward? Were these resources adequate?

28.2 Create a list of interventions found at your place of work or the literature and rate them from 1 (worst) to 5 (best) in their effectiveness to prevent harm from workplace violence.

- What are the top five interventions that you believe are the most successful in reducing violence and harm from violence in healthcare?
- Can you identify high reliability principles used in the interventions?

LEARNING ACTIVITY IMPLEMENTATION

Students will benefit the most from these learning activities when they do them in a group.

For Exercise 28.1, students discuss their personal experience with workplace violence as a healthcare professional in small groups. Students should discuss what happened, their reaction, what provoked the violent act, and what resources were accessible in the aftermath of the violent event.

For Exercise 28.2, students should create a list of interventions in the workplace or from the literature and rate them in effectiveness to prevent harm from workplace violence. Students should include application of high reliability principles.

These exercises can be accomplished in a discussion occurring in the physical classroom, in an online synchronous classroom, or in a facilitator-prompted course-platform-based discussion board. Also, facilitators may consider these exercises as a graded paper or student presentation to the class.

STUDENT EVALUATION

Facilitators should evaluate the following:

28.1 Did the student's discussion of their personal experience with workplace violence include what happened, their reaction, provocation of the event, and accessible resources post event?

28.2 Was the student able to create a list of effective interventions to reduce violence and harm from violence in healthcare?

CHAPTER 29

INTRODUCTION OF HIGH RELIABILITY TO FRONTLINE STAFF: CREATING A VIRTUAL RESOURCE TOOLKIT

In this chapter, students will learn about how high reliability principles can be used to build a highly reliable team that is foundational in an HRO. Students will learn about how building a resource toolkit can foster an environment of high reliability and promote growth within a culture of safety.

Learning Objective

Explore how to leverage high reliability principles on an organization-level interprofessional team to build a resource toolkit to foster a culture of patient safety.

Learning Activity 29.1: Apply High Reliability Principles to Solve Organizational Team Quality and Safety Challenges

Learning Activity Objectives

29.1 Use HRO characteristics to design a healthcare organization interprofessional resource toolkit that promotes a culture of safety (*applying*).

29.2 Select an interprofessional team where application of high reliability could fulfill an organizational strategic initiative of nurturing a culture of high reliability and patient safety (*applying*).

29.3 Design an interprofessional project plan to develop an organizational resource toolkit using high reliability principles to nurture a culture of high reliability and patient safety (*creating*).

Preparation

Prior to completion of the learning activity, students should:

- Read Chapter 29.
- Identify an interprofessional team to apply high reliability to fulfill an organizational strategic initiative.
- Read "Development and Expression of a High-Reliability Organization" at https://doi.org/10.1056/CAT.21.0314.

Instructions

29.1 Identify an organizational culture of safety strategic initiative that could be affected by an interprofessional resource toolkit using high reliability principles.

29.2 Using knowledge of high reliability principles, explain which high reliability principles are relevant in addressing the strategic initiative and why (see Table 29.1).

Answer Example:

TABLE 29.1 APPLYING HIGH RELIABILITY PRINCIPLES TO A STRATEGIC INITIATIVE

Strategic Initiative	Principle 1 Preoccupation With Failure	Principle 2 Reluctance to Simplify	Principle 3 Sensitivity to Operations	Principle 4 Commitment to Resilience	Principle 5 Deference to Expertise
Commission team to fulfill organizational strategic initiative of nurturing a culture of high reliability and patient safety within the organization with a primary objective of providing strategic guidance for organizational priorities related to patient safety education development.	Identify barriers to learning and access to resources.	Perform a needs analysis to assess current knowledge, skills, and attitudes of the frontline staff about concepts related to patient safety and high reliability.	Determine whether frontline staff could locate high reliability and patient safety resources within the organization.	Encourage interprofessional education for a culture of continuous learning and support.	Interprofessional team members act as subject matter experts and include physicians, patient safety specialists, quality and analytics staff, all levels of nurse leaders from both inpatient and ambulatory services, patient family advisors, and directors and leaders from the offices of regulatory compliance and quality and risk.

29.3 Design an interprofessional resource toolkit project plan using the principles of high reliability to meet an organizational culture of safety strategic initiative. There are nine sections to complete this activity (see Figure 29.1).

1. Describe the quality/safety project.
2. Identify the project deliverables.
3. List the baseline measures related to the project.
4. Complete the project plan charter form.
5. List steps or approaches/ideas on how you, as the team leader, would ensure integration of the high reliability principles into the solution(s).
6. Describe any risks or threats to the project.
7. Briefly describe a communication plan for the project.
8. Briefly describe a training plan for the project.
9. Briefly describe how you would evaluate the project's success.

CHAPTER 29 INTRODUCTION OF HIGH RELIABILITY TO FRONTLINE STAFF: CREATING A VIRTUAL RESOURCE TOOLKIT

Potential Project Name/Title		Date	
Requested by		Charter Prepared by	

Background & Business Need: State the business problem/issue to solve or what opportunity exists to improve a business function. What is the current state? Narrative background with drivers for the project.

Project Scope Statement: Summarize the purpose and the intent of the project and describe what the customer (or you) envisions will be delivered.

Project Objectives/Deliverables: Outline the high-level objectives for the project. What will exist when the project is complete? Include the benefits of the project, including how the project will benefit the customers or stakeholders.

Boundaries: What will _not_ be included in this project?

Assumptions: What assumptions were made when conceiving this project?

External Dependencies: Note any major external (to the project) dependencies the project must rely upon for success, such as specific technologies, third-party vendors, development partners, or other business relationships. Also identify any other related projects or initiatives.

Project Risks: List any known risks for the project that could impact the success of the project or should be considered when planning. Include risk of change management. Does the value of this project ultimately depend on people changing their work or behavior? Identify risks facing this project or organization if the people side of the project is poorly manned.

Key Stakeholders: List the key stakeholders for the project. Stakeholders are individuals, groups, or organizations that are actively involved in a project, are affected by its outcome, or can influence its outcome. Indicate their role or interest in the project. These stakeholders (or representatives) MAY be invited to participate in a project kickoff session but do not necessarily need to be on the project team. Whose day-to-day work will be impacted by raw processes (systems, tools, job roles, organization structure, etc.) as an outcome or deliverable of this project?

Stakeholder/Stakeholder Group	Role in Project or Impacted by This Project

Required Resources: Identify the known resources that management is willing to commit to the project at this time. Human resources includes key individuals, teams, organizations, subcontractors or vendors, and support functions. This is not the place for the detailed team staff roster for individual names. Identify critical skill sets that team members must have. Other resources could include funding, computers, other equipment, physical facilities such as buildings and rooms, hardware devices, software tools, and training. What level of change management involvement is expected for this project? (e.g., separate change management team, change management representation on the core team or individual team).

Requested Timeline/Milestones: Include end and start dates and key milestones.

Figure 29.1 Nine-step project plan template.

LEARNING ACTIVITY IMPLEMENTATION

Students will benefit the most from these learning activities when they do them in a group of four or five students.

For Exercise 29.1, students identify an organizational culture of safety strategic initiative opportunity that could be affected by an interprofessional resource toolkit using high reliability principles. The opportunity can be from their organization or from the literature.

For Exercise 29.2, students apply high reliability principles to design an interprofessional resource toolkit that addresses the organizational strategic initiative. Using knowledge of high reliability principles, explain which high reliability principles are relevant in addressing the strategic initiative and why.

For Exercise 29.3, students should design a project plan for an interprofessional team resource toolkit to address an organizational culture of safety strategic initiative opportunity identified in Exercise 29.1. The nine-step project plan template is shown in Figure 29.1.

These exercises can be accomplished in a discussion occurring in the physical classroom, in an online synchronous classroom, or in a facilitator-prompted course-platform-based discussion board. Also, facilitators may consider these exercises as a graded paper or student presentation to the class.

STUDENT EVALUATION

Facilitators should evaluate the following:

29.1 Did the student identify an organizational culture of safety strategic initiative that could be affected by an interprofessional resource toolkit using high reliability principles?

29.2 Was the student able to identify an organizational culture of safety strategic initiative where an interprofessional resource toolkit could impact the culture of safety through the use of high reliability principles? Was the student able to link how the resource toolkit connects with each high reliability principle?

29.3 Did the student design an interprofessional resource toolkit project plan using the principles of high reliability to meet an organizational culture of safety strategic initiative?

PART IX

TRANSLATION INTO PRACTICE SUMMATIVE ASSESSMENT

Learning Objective
Examine how high reliability principles are translated into practice.

Contents
Summative Assessment: Translation Into Practice............140

Supplemental Facilitator Resources and Readings..........144

SUMMATIVE ASSESSMENT: TRANSLATION INTO PRACTICE

This summative course assessment evaluates student learning at the end of the course. This assessment may be used as a comprehensive measure of student understanding and ability to translate EBP, change management, and high reliability principles to practice.

Learning Objective

Examine how high reliability principles are translated into practice.

Summative Assessment Learning Activity: Translate Evidence-Based Practice, Change Management, and High Reliability Principles to Practice

Summative Assessment Learning Activity Objectives

SA.1 Show an EBP model and a change management model (*understanding*).

SA.2 Summarize characteristics of EBP process, change management, and high reliability principles in one of the provided examples (*understanding*).

SA.3 Apply characteristics of the EBP process, change management, and high reliability principles to a student-selected clinical practice problem (*applying*).

Preparation

Prior to completion of the learning activity, students should:

- Read chapters within the textbook that describe a process for improvement of interest.

Instructions

SA.1 Show an EBP model and a change management model. Choose one chapter from the book describing a project that led to an improvement. Using selected EBP and change management models, identify steps of the EBP process and change management process described in the chapter. The EBP Worksheet (Appendix A in this facilitator guide) may be useful for students to complete this exercise. Answer the following questions to evaluate the translation-into-practice example:

- How did the project use data to identify the need for change or define the problem?
- How was literature used to explain the rationale for the intervention?
- Is the intervention based on a theory?
- How did the authors obtain buy-in from stakeholders?
- Was there any evidence of resistance to change?
- How was resistance to change addressed?
- How was data collected and analyzed?
- Was a tool used for data collection?
- Is there a plan for sustainability?

SA.2 Summarize characteristics and use of high reliability principles within the aforementioned translation-into-practice example. "High Reliability Organizations: A Quick Guide for Frontline Application," Appendix B in this facilitator guide, may be a useful tool to students for completing this exercise.

SA.3 Identify a problem from your own practice and integrate EBP steps, change management principles, and high reliability principles to create a sustainable practice change. Create a basic proposal to describe your plan. Include the following:

- Background and significance of the problem
- Problem statement
- Objectives and aims of the project, intervention description
- Methodology
- Proposed intervention
- Setting and participants
- Proposed outcome measures and evaluation
- Data collection plan
- Data analysis plan

Include a description of a tool or method of high reliability.

Include a description of a principle of change management.

SUMMATIVE ASSESSMENT LEARNING ACTIVITY IMPLEMENTATION

Students should complete the summative assessment learning activity exercises individually.

For SA.1, students select one of the clinical translations-into-practice examples in the textbook. The student should be able to identify EBP process steps along with change management processes. The EBP Worksheet (Appendix A in this facilitator guide) may be helpful for students completing this exercise.

For SA.2, students identify characteristics and use of high reliability principles within the selected translation-into-practice example. The student should be able to trace how high reliability principles were translated into practice. "High Reliability Organizations: A Quick Guide for Frontline Application," Appendix B in this facilitator guide, may be helpful for students to use to complete this exercise.

For SA.3, each student prepares a draft proposal for a sustainable practice change. The proposal is comprehensive in nature. Facilitators should guide students to translate high reliability principles discussed throughout the course into clinical practice. Students should integrate EBP steps, change management principles, and high reliability principles to create a sustainable practice change.

These exercises can be accomplished in a discussion in the physical classroom, in an online synchronous classroom, or in a facilitator-prompted course-platform-based discussion board. Facilitators may consider Exercises SA.1 and SA.2 as a presentation to the class. Exercise SA.3 is intended as a graded paper with sources, in lieu of a final exam.

STUDENT EVALUATION

Facilitators should evaluate the following:

SA.1 Was the student able to identify steps of the EBP process and change management process in a translation-into-practice example?

SA.2 Was the student able to identify characteristics and use of high reliability principles in a translation-into-practice example?

SA.3 Was the student able to translate EBP, change management, and high reliability principles to draft a proposal for a sustainable practice change?

SUPPLEMENTAL FACILITATOR RESOURCES AND READINGS

UNIT 3, PART I

CHAPTER 1

Conklin, T. *Pre-accident investigation podcast.* https://preaccidentpodcast.podbean.com/

Dekker, S. (2025). *What is safety differently?* https://sidneydekker.com/

Kuhlman, J. & Roncska, R. (2024). *High reliability healthcare: Applying the secrets of the nuclear navy to save patient lives.* Ballast Books. http://www.ballastbooks.com/

Myers, G. & Sutcliffe, K. (2022). High reliability organizing in healthcare: still a long way left to go. *BMJ Quality and Safety,* 31, 845-848. https://doi.org/10.1136/bmjqs-2021-014141

Weick, K. E., & Sutcliffe, K. M. (2015). *Managing the unexpected: Sustaining performance in a complex world.* (3rd ed.). John Wiley & Sons.

CHAPTER 2

Armstrong, G., & Sherwood, G. (2020). Patient safety. In J. F. Giddens (Eds.) *Concepts for nursing practice* (pp. 434–442). Elsevier.

Barnsteiner, J. (2022). Safety. In G. Sherwood & J. Barnsteiner (Eds.), *Quality and safety in nursing: A competency approach to improving outcomes* (pp. 149–170). Wiley-Blackwell.

Reason, J. (2000). Human error: Models and management. *British Medical Journal, 320*(7237), 768–770. https://doi.org/10.1136/bmj.320.7237.768

Sherwood, G. (2022). Driving forces for quality and safety: Changing mindsets to improve healthcare. In G. Sherwood & J. Barnsteiner (Eds.), *Quality and safety in nursing: A competency approach to improving outcomes* (pp. 3–21). Wiley-Blackwell.

CHAPTER 3

Al-Amin, M., Schiaffino, M. K., Park, S., & Harman, J. (2018). Sustained hospital performance on consumer assessment of healthcare providers and system survey measures. What are the determinants? *Foundation of the American College of Healthcare Executives, 36*(1), 15–28. https://doi.org/10.1097/JHM-D-16-00006

Ellenbogen, M. I., Ellenbogen, P. M., Rim, N., & Brotman, D. J. (2022). Characterizing the relationship between hospital Google star ratings, Hospital Consumer Assessment of Healthcare Providers and Systems (HCAHPS) scores, and quality. *Journal of Patient Experience, 9.* https://doi.org/10.1177/23743735221092604

Makic, M. B. F., & Granger, B. B. (2019). Deimplementation in clinical practice. What are we waiting for? *AACN Advanced Critical Care, 30*(3), 282–286. https://doi.org/10.4037/aacnacc2019607

Padula, W. V., Lee, K. K. H., & Pronovost, P. J. (2021). Using economic evaluation to illustrate value of care for improving patient safety and quality: Choosing the right method. *Journal of Patient Safety, 17*(6), e568–e574. https://doi.org/10.1097/PTS.0000000000000410

Sutcliffe, K. M. (2023). Building cultures of high reliability: Lessons from the high reliability organization paradigm. *Anesthesiology Clinics, 41*(4), 707–717. https://doi.org/10.1016/j.anclin.2023.03.012

CHAPTER 4

Bellot, J. (2011). Defining and assessing organizational culture. *Nursing Forum, 46*(1), 29–37. https://doi.org/10.1111/j.1744-6198.2010.00207.x

Cartland, J., Green, M., Kamm, D., Halfer, D., Brisk, M. A., & Wheeler, D. (2022). Measuring psychological safety and local learning to enable high reliability organizational change. *BMJ Open Quality, 11*(4), e001757. https://doi.org/10.1136/bmjoq-2021-001757

Edmondson, A. C. (2019). *The fearless organization: Creating psychological safety in the workplace for learning, innovation, and growth.* Wiley.

Gallo, A. (2023, February 15). What is psychological safety? *Harvard Business Review.* https://hbr.org/2023/02/what-is-psychological-safety

Ito, A., Sato, K., Yumoto, Y., Sasaki, M., & Ogata, Y. (2022). A concept analysis of psychological safety: Further understanding for application to health care. *Nursing Open, 9*(1), 467–489. https://doi.org/10.1002/nop2.1086

CHAPTER 5

Edmondson, A. (2019). *The fearless organization: Creating psychological safety in the workplace for learning, innovation, and growth.* Wiley.

Ford, J. L. (2018). Revisiting high-reliability organizing: Obstacles to safety and resilience. *Corporate Communications: An International Journal, 23*(2), 197–211. https://doi.org/10.1108/CCIJ-04-2017-0034

Omidi, L., Karimi, H., Pilbeam, C., Mousavi, S., & Moradi, G. (2023). Exploring the relationships among safety leadership, safety climate, psychological contract of safety, risk perception, safety compliance, and safety outcomes. *Frontiers in Public Health, 11*, 1235214. https://doi.org/10.3389/fpubh.2023.1235214

Weick, K. E., & Sutcliffe, K. M. (2015). *Managing the unexpected: Sustaining performance in a complex world* (3rd ed.). Wiley.

CHAPTER 6

Jack, L. (2021). Advancing health equity, eliminating health disparities, and improving population health. *Preventing Chronic Disease, 18*, 210264. http://dx.doi.org/10.5888/pcd18.210264

Moy, E., Hausmann, L. R., & Clancy, C. M. (2022). From HRO to HERO: Making health equity a core system capability. *American Journal of Medical Quality, 37*(1), 81-83. https://doi.org/10.1097/JMQ.0000000000000020

Togioka, B. M., Duvivier D., & Young, E. (2025, January). Diversity and discrimination in health care. *StatPearls.* https://www.ncbi.nlm.nih.gov/books/NBK568721/

World Health Organization. (n.d.). *Health equity.* https://www.who.int/health-topics/health-equity#tab=tab_1

UNIT 3, PART II

CHAPTER 7

CMS. (n.d). *Guidance for performing failure mode and effects analysis with performance improvement projects.* https://www.cms.gov/Medicare/Provider-Enrollment-and-Certification/QAPI/Downloads/GuidanceForFMEA.pdf

Pidgeon, N. (2010). *Systems thinking, culture of reliability and safety. Civil Engineering and Environmental Systems, 27*(3), 211–217. https://www.icesi.edu.co/blogs/pslunes122/files/2012/08/Systems-thinking-culture-of-reliability-and-safety1.pdf

CHAPTER 8

Almansour, H. (2024). Barriers preventing the reporting of incidents and near misses among healthcare professionals. *Journal of Health Management, 26*(1), 78–84. https://doi.org/10.1177/09720634231167031

The Joint Commission. (2018). *Developing a reporting culture: Learning from close calls and hazardous conditions.* https://www.jointcommission.org/-/media/tjc/documents/resources/patient-safety-topics/sentinel-event/sea_60_reporting_culture_final.pdf?db=web&hash=5AB072026CAAF4711FCDC343701B0159

Uibu, E., Põlluste, K., Lember, M., & Kangasniemi, M. (2020). Reporting and responding to patient safety incidents based on data from hospitals' reporting systems: A systematic review. *Journal of Hospital Administration, 9*(2), 22-32. https://doi.org/10.5430/jha.v9n2p22

Woo, M. W. J., & Avery, M. J. (2021). Nurses' experiences in voluntary error reporting: An integrative literature review. *International Journal of Nursing Sciences, 8*(4), 453–469. https://doi.org/10.1016/j.ijnss.2021.07.004

UNIT 3, PART III

CHAPTER 9

Dekker, S. (2011). *Patient safety: A human factors approach*. CRC Press.

Holden, R. J., Carayon, P., Gurses, A. P., Hoonakker, P., Hundt, A. S., Ozok, A. A., & Rivera-Rodriguez, A. J. (2013). SEIPS 2.0: a human factors framework for studying and improving the work of healthcare professionals and patients. *Ergonomics, 56*(11), 1669–1686. https://doi.org/10.1080/00140139.2013.838643

Marriott, R. D. (2018). Process mapping–The foundation for effective quality improvement. *Current Problems in Pediatric and Adolescent Health Care, 48*(7), 177–181. https://doi.org/10.1016/j.cppeds.2018.08.010

Weaver, B. W., Gannon, P. R., & Mumma, J. M. (2024). Improving patient safety by design: The role of human factors engineering. In C. A. Oster & J. S. Braaten (Eds.) *The nexus between nursing and patient safety* (pp. 241–257). Springer Nature.

CHAPTER 10

Institute for Healthcare Improvement. (n.d.). *RCA²: Improving root cause analyses and actions to prevent harm*. https://www.ihi.org/resources/tools/rca2-improving-root-cause-analyses-and-actions-prevent-harm#:~:text=This%20tool%20describes%20best%20practices%20for%20conducting%20a,actions%20will%20have%20the%20strongest%20effect%20for%20succes

Maternity & Newborn Safety Investigations. (2024). *Why it made sense at the time: Local rationality questions for healthcare investigations*. https://www.mnsi.org.uk/news/local-rationality-questions-for-healthcare-investigations/

National Patient Safety Foundation. (2016). *RCA² Improving root cause analysis and actions to prevent harm*. https://www.med.unc.edu/ihqi/files/2018/07/RCA2-National-Patient-Safety-Foundation.pdf

Sampson, P., Back, J., & Drage, S. (2021). Systems-based models for investigating patient safety incidents. *BJA Education, 21*(8), 307–313. https://doi.org/10.1016/j.bjae.2021.03.004

CHAPTER 11

Dekker, S. (2013). *Second victim: Error, guilt, trauma, and resilience*. Chapman & Hall/CRC.

Dekker, S. (2018). *Just Culture: Restoring trust and accountability in your organization* (3rd ed.). Chapman & Hall/CRC.

Marx, D. (2009). *Whack-a-mole: The price we pay for expecting perfection*. By Your Side Studios.

Marx, D. (2019). Reckless homicide at Vanderbilt? A Just Culture analysis. https://www.linkedin.com/pulse/reckless-homicide-vanderbilt-just-culture-analysis-david-marx/

Ozeke, O., Ozeke, V., Coskun, O., & Budakoglu, I. I. (2019). Second victims in health care: Current perspectives. *Advances in Medical Education & Practice, 10*, 593–603. https://doi.org/10.2147/AMEP.S185912

Restorative Just Culture Checklist. https://safetydifferently.com/restorative-just-culture-checklist/restorativejustculturechecklist-2/

UNIT 3, PART IV

CHAPTER 12

Hravnak, M., Pellathy, T., Chen, L., Dubrawski, A., Wertz, A., Clermont, G., & Pinsky, M. R. (2018). A call to alarms: Current state and future directions in the battle against alarm fatigue. *Journal of Electrocardiology, 51*(6S), pp. S44–S48. https://www.ncbi.nlm.nih.gov/pmc/articles/PMC6263784/pdf/nihms-1502834.pdf

Woo, M., & Bacon, O. (2020, March 13). Alarm fatigue. In K. K. Hall, S. Shoemaker-Hunt, L. Hoffman, et al. *Making healthcare safer III: A critical analysis of existing and emerging patient safety practices*. Agency for Healthcare Research and Quality. https://www.ncbi.nlm.nih.gov/books/NBK555522/

CHAPTER 13

Englebright, J. (2019). *Ideal nursing workflows to support the development of information technology solutions*. Sigma Repository. https://www.sigmarepository.org/gen_sub_csm/30/

Fraczkowski, D., Matson, J., & Lopez, K. D. (2020). Nurse workarounds in the electronic health record: An integrative review. *Journal of the American Medical Informatics Association, 27*(7), 1149-1165. https://doi.org/10.1093/jamia/ocaa050

Human Factors Engineering. PSNet [internet]. Rockville (MD): Agency for Healthcare Research and Quality, US Department of Health and Human Services. 2019. https://psnet.ahrq.gov/primer/human-factors-engineering

Soong, C., & Shojania, K. G. (2020). Education as a low-value improvement intervention: Often necessary but rarely sufficient. *BMJ Quality & Safety, 29*(5), 353-357. https://doi.org/10.1136/bmjqs-2019-010411

CHAPTER 14

Goldenhar, L. M., Brady, P. W., Sutcliffe, K. M., & Muething, S. E. (2013). Huddling for high reliability and situation awareness. *BMJ Quality & Safety, 22*(11), 899–906. https://doi.org/10.1136/bmjqs-2012-001467

Merchant, N.B., O'Neal, J., Montoya, A., Cox, G.R., & Murray, J.S. (2023). Creating a process for the implementation of tiered huddles in a Veterans Affairs medical center. *Military Medicine, 188*(5-6), 901–906. https://doi.org/10.1093/milmed/usac073

UNIT 3, PART V

CHAPTER 15

Brooks, A., Fitzpatrick, S., & Dunlap, E. (2022). Creating a culture of teamwork through the use of the TeamSTEPPS framework: A review of the literature and considerations for nurse practitioners. *Journal of Leadership Education, 21*(1), 155–162. https://doi.org/10.12806/V21/I1/R11

Edmondson, A. C. (2012). *Teaming: How organizations learn, innovate, and compete in the knowledge economy*. Wiley.

Rosen, M. A., DiazGranados, D., Dietz, A. S., Benishek, L. E., Thompson, D., Pronovost, P. J., & Weaver, S. J. (2018). Teamwork in healthcare: Key discoveries enabling safer, high-quality care. *American Psychologist, 73*(4), 433–450. https://doi.org/10.1037/amp0000298.

CHAPTER 16

Agency for Healthcare Research and Quality. (2023, March). *Guide to patient and family engagement in hospital quality and safety*. https://www.ahrq.gov/patient-safety/patients-families/engagingfamilies/index.html

Agency for Clinical Innovation. (2019). *Patient experience and consumer engagement—A guide to build co-design capability*. https://aci.health.nsw.gov.au/data/assets/pdf_file/0013/502240/ACI-Guide-build-codesign-capability.pdf

McGowan, D., Morley, C., Hansen, E., Shaw, K., & Winzenberg, T. (2024). Experiences of participants in the co-design of a community-based health service for people with high healthcare service use. *BMC Health Services Research, 24*(1), 339. https://doi.org/10.1186/s12913-024-10788-5

Newman, B., Joseph, K., Chauhan, A., Seale, H., Li, J., Manias, E., Walton, M., Mears, S., Jones, B., & Harrison, R. (2021). Do patient engagement interventions work for all patients? A systematic review and realist synthesis of interventions to enhance patient safety. *Health Expectations, 24*(6), 1905–1923. https://doi.org/10.1111/hex.13343

CHAPTER 17

Caporale-Berkowitz, N., & Friedman, S. D. (2018). How peer coaching can make work less lonely. *Harvard Business Review*. https://hbr.org/2018/10/how-peer-coaching-can-make-work-less-lonely

Kotter, J. (1995, March-April). Leading change: why transformation efforts fail. *Harvard Business Review*. https://hbr.org/1995/03/leading-change-why-transformation-efforts-fail-2

Pfeifer, L., Vessey, J., Cazzell, M., Ponte, P. R., & Geyer, D. (2023). Relationships among psychological safety, the principles of high reliability, and safety reporting intentions in pediatric nursing. *Journal of Pediatric Nursing, 73*, 130–136. https://doi.org/10.1016/j.pedn.2023.09.001

UNIT 3, PART VI

CHAPTER 18

National Academies of Sciences, Engineering, and Medicine. (2019). *Taking action against clinician burnout: A systems approach to professional well-being*. The National Academies Press. https://doi.org/10.17226/25521

Rushton, C. H. (2023). Transforming moral suffering by cultivating moral resilience and ethical practice. *American Journal of Critical Care, 32*(4), 238–248. https://doi.org/10.4037/ajcc2023207

CHAPTER 19

International Nursing Association for Clinical Simulation and Learning. https://www.inacsl.org/

Lamé, G., & Dixon-Woods, M. (2020). Using clinical simulation to study how to improve quality and safety in healthcare. *BMJ Simulation & Technology Enhanced Learning, 6*(2), 87-94. https://doi.org/10.1136/bmjstel-2018-000370

CHAPTER 20

Granitto, M., Linenfelser, P., Hursey, R., Parsons, M., & Norton, C. (2020). Empowering nurses to activate the rapid response team. *Nursing, 50*(6), 52-57. https://doi.org/10.1097/01.NURSE.0000662356.08413.90

Williams, K-L., Rideout, J., Pritchett-Kelly, J., McDonald, M., Mullins-Richards, M., & Dubrowski, A. (2016, December). Mock code: A code blue scenario requested by and developed for registered nurses. *Cureus, 8*(12), e938. http://doi.org/10.7759/cureus.938

Won, Y. H., & Kang, J. (2022). Development of a comprehensive model for the role of the rapid response team nurse. *Intensive & Critical Care Nursing, 68*, 103136. https://doi.org/10.1016/j.iccn.2021.103136

CHAPTER 21

Black, J. S. (2014). *It starts with one: Changing individuals changes organizations* (3rd ed.). Pearson Education.

Dekker, S. (2017). *Just Culture—Restoring trust and accountability in your organization* (3rd ed.). CRC Press/ Taylor & Francis Group.

Rodriguez, R., Hambley, C., & Wisner, K. (2024). Taking the fear out of peer feedback: A brain-friendly peer feedback program. *Journal of Nursing Administration, 54*(1), 40–46. https://doi.org/10.1097/NNA.0000000000001375

UNIT 3, PART VII

CHAPTER 22

Auraaen, A., L. Slawomirski, L., & Klazinga, N. (2018), The economics of patient safety in primary and ambulatory care: Flying blind. *OECD Health Working Papers*, No. 106. OECD Publishing. https://doi.org/10.1787/baf425ad-en

Gaguski, M. E., & Nguyen, H. T. (2016). An interdisciplinary approach to the development and implementation of electronic treatment orders in a medical oncology department. *Clinical Journal of Oncology Nursing, 20*(4), 371–373. https://www.ons.org/articles/interdisciplinary-approach-development-and-implementation-electronic-treatment-orders

Siaki, L., Patrician, P. A., Loan, L. A., Matlock, A.M., Start, R. E., & McCarthy, M. S. (2022). Improving 9.5 million lives: Pilot testing ambulatory care nurse-sensitive quality indicators. *Journal of Nursing Administration, 52*(11), 613–619. https://doi.org/10.1097/NNA.0000000000001218

CHAPTER 23

American Nurses Credentialing Center. (n.d.). *Magnet Model – Creating a Magnet Culture*. https://www.nursingworld.org/organizational-programs/magnet/magnet-model/

McGinnis, J., Aquino-Maneja, E., Geloso, K., Zaragoza, C., Spicer, J., & Kawar, L. N. (2024). Regional transformation: An integrated system's approach to Magnet designation utilizing high-reliability organization implementation strategies. *Journal of Nursing Care Quality, 39*(4), 345–353. https://doi.org/10.1097/NCQ.0000000000000782

Rodríguez-García, M. C., Márquez-Hernández, V. V., Belmonte-García, T., Gutiérrez-Puertas, L., & Granados-Gámez, G. (2020). How Magnet hospital status affects nurses, patients, and organizations: A systematic review. *American Journal of Nursing, 120*(7), 28–38. https://doi.org/10.1097/01.NAJ.0000681648.48249.16

CHAPTER 24

American Nurses Association. (June 1, 2023). *What is evidence-based practice in nursing?* https://www.nursingworld.org/content-hub/resources/workplace/evidence-based-practice-in-nursing/

Associates in Process Improvement. (n.d.). *How to improve: Model for improvement.* Institute for Healthcare Improvement. https://www.ihi.org/resources/how-improve-model-improvement

Kim, H. J., Kawar, L. N., Rondinelli, J., Aquino-Maneja, E. M., McGinnis, J. A., Scruth, E., Torgrimson-Ojerio, B., D'Alfonso, J., Watkins, A. M., & Doulaveris, P. (2024). The role of the nurse scientist and nursing research within a national integrated health care system. *Nursing Administration Quarterly, 48*(3), 237–247. https://doi.org/10.1097/NAQ.0000000000000644

Lai, M.M. (2021). Why nursing research matters. *Journal of Nursing Administration, 51*(5), 235-236. https://doi.org/10.1097/NNA.0000000000001005

Mulkey, M. A. (2021). Engaging bedside nurse in research and quality improvement. *Journal for Nurses in Professional Development, 37*(3), 138–142. https://doi.org/10.1097/NND.0000000000000732

CHAPTER 25

Rosário, M., & Fonseca, A. C. (2022). Incorporating quality improvement projects into stroke care and research. *Stroke, 53*(3), e118–e121. https://doi.org/10.1161/STROKEAHA.121.038204

UNIT 3, PART VIII

CHAPTER 26

Benton, D.C., Alexander, M., Fotsch, R., & Livanos, N. (2020, August 12). Lessons learned and insights gained: A regulatory analysis of the impacts, challenges, and responses to COVID-19. *OJIN: The Online Journal of Issues in Nursing, 25*(3). https://doi.org/10.3912/OJIN.Vol25No03PPT51

Doos, D., Hughes, A. M., Pham, T., Barach, P., Bona, A., Falvo, L., Moore, M., Cooper, Dylan D., & Ahmed, R. (2024). Frontline health care workers' COVID-19 infection contamination risks: A human factors and risk analysis study of personal protective equipment. *American Journal of Medical Quality 39*(1), 4–13. https://doi.org/10.1097/JMQ.0000000000000159

Gregory, D. D., Stichler, J. F., & Zborowsky, T. (2022). Adapting and creating healing environments: lessons nurses have learned from the COVID-19 pandemic. *Nurse Leader, 20*(2), 201-207. https://doi.org/10.1016/j.mnl.2021.10.013

Mumma, J. M., Durso, F. T., Casanova, L. M., Erukunuakpor, K., Kraft, C. S., Ray, S. M., Shane, A. L., Walsh, V. L., Shah, P. Y., Zimring, C., DuBose, J., & Jacob, J. T. (2019). Variability in the duration and thoroughness of hand hygiene. *Clinical Infectious Diseases, 69*(Suppl. 3), S221–S223. https://doi.org/10.1093/cid/ciz612

CHAPTER 27

Guttman, O. T., Lazzara, E. H., Keebler, J. R., Webster, K. L., Gisick, L. M., & Baker, A. L. (2023). Closed-loop communication in interprofessional emergency teams: A cross-sectional observation study on the use of closed-loop communication among anesthesia personnel. *Journal of Patient Safety, 19*(2), 93–99. https://doi.org/10.1097/PTS.0000000000001098

Sanchez, J. A., & Barach, P. R. (2012). High reliability organizations and surgical microsystems: Re-engineering surgical care. *Surgical Clinics of North America, 92*(1), 1–14. https://doi.org/10.1016/j.suc.2011.12.005

Stucky, C. H., Wymer, J. A., & House, S. (2022). Nurse leaders: Transforming interprofessional relationships to bridge healthcare quality and safety. *Nurse Leader*, *20*(4), 375-380. https://doi.org/10.1016/j.mnl.2021.12.003

CHAPTER 28

American Society for Health Care Risk Management. (n.d*.*). *Health care facility workplace violence risk assessment toolkit*. https://www.ashrm.org/resources/workplace_violence

O'Brien, C. J., van Zundert, A. A., & Barach, P. R. (2024). The growing burden of workplace violence against healthcare workers: Trends in prevalence, risk factors, consequences, and prevention–a narrative review. *EClinicalMedicine*, *72*. https://doi.org/10.1016/j.eclinm.2024.102641

CHAPTER 29

Heron, L., & Bruk-Lee, V. (2020). When empowered nurses are under stress: Understanding the impact on attitudes and behaviours. *Stress and Health*, *36*(2), 147–159. https://doi.org/10.1002/smi.2905

Phillips, R. A., Schwartz, R. L., Sostman, H. D., & Boom, M. L. (2021). Development and expression of a high-reliability organization. *NEJM Catalyst Innovations in Care Delivery*, *2*(12). https://doi.org/10.1056/CAT.21.0314

Veazie, S., Peterson, K., & Bourne, D. (2019). *Evidence brief: Implementation of high reliability organization principles*. https://www.hsrd.research.va.gov/publications/esp/high-reliability-org-supplemental.pdf

UNIT 3, PART IX

SUMMATIVE ASSESSMENT COURSE ASSESSMENT

Cullen, L., Hanrahan, K., Farrington, M., Tucker, S., & Edmonds, C. (2022). *Evidence-based practice in action: Comprehensive strategies, tools, and tips from the University of Iowa Hospitals and Clinics*, (2nd ed.). Sigma Theta Tau International.

Houser, J., & Oman, K. (Eds.). (2011*)*. *Evidence-based practice: An implementation guide for healthcare organizations*. Jones & Bartlett.

Mazurek-Melnyk, B,. & Fineholt-Overholt, E. (2022). *Evidence-based practice in nursing & healthcare: A guide to best practice* (5th ed.). Wolters Kluwer.

APPENDICES

Contents

Appendix A: EBP Worksheet 153

Appendix B: High Reliability Organizations: A Quick Guide for
              Frontline Application 156

EBP WORKSHEET

Appendix A: EBP Worksheet

Project Title		
Name (Stakeholders)	Unit	Title
Unit Manager's Name and Work		

Problem Identified: What is a problem you see at your work? NDNQI, such as PI, Fall, CAUTI? What is your current number? How are you able to obtain that?

Patient Outcome: What is the patient outcome expected to improve? How are you going to measure?

Process Outcome: What is the process outcome to assess effectiveness of your project? How are you going to measure?

PICO Concepts for Developing a Purpose Statement

Patient Population

Clinical **P**roblem or Condition (include numbers to support, such as fall rate or CAUTI rate)

Interventions

What do you want to implement?

How do you want to implement?

Comparison

Anticipated **O**utcomes (Process Outcome and Patient Outcome)

Patient Outcome

Process Outcome

Next Steps

Your Work Plan/Next Steps

-
-
-

HIGH RELIABILITY ORGANIZATIONS: A QUICK GUIDE FOR FRONTLINE APPLICATION

Objectives for the user of this guide:

- Understand the concept of high reliability organizations (HROs) and their application to patient safety.
- Explain the five principles of HROs as described by Weick and Sutcliffe.
- Apply the principles to your work area by discussing key questions.
- Use a guide to identify a process in your work area that requires high reliability.
- Use a guide to analyze and improve the process by using high reliability techniques.

What Are High Reliability Organizations (HROs)?

HROs are those that are high risk, dynamic, turbulent, and potentially hazardous, yet operate nearly error free. Examples include aviation, nuclear engineering, defense operations, and acute care hospitals.

How do HROs stay error free?

- HROs recognize that small things that go wrong are often early warning signs of trouble. The warning signs are the "red flags" that provide insight into the health of the whole system.
- HROs value near misses as indicators of early trouble and are acted on to prevent future failure. Near misses are not seen as an indicator of system success.
- HROs are innovative and creative, and they value input from all corners of the organization.
- HROs recognize the value of preparing for the unexpected and the unknown. Failures rarely occur if they are expected.

The five principles of HROs follow:

- Preoccupation with failure: HROs are preoccupied with all failures, especially small ones. Small things that go wrong are often early warning signals of deepening trouble and give insight into the health of the whole system. But we have a tendency to ignore or overlook our failures (which suggest we are not competent) and focus on our successes (which suggest we are competent).
- Reluctance to simplify: HROs restrain their temptation to simplify through diverse checks and balances, adversarial reviews, and the cultivation of multiple perspectives.
- Sensitivity to operations: HROs make strong responses to weak signals (indications that something might be amiss). Everyone values organizing to maintain situational awareness.
- Commitment to resilience: HROs pay close attention to their capability to improvise and act—without knowing in advance what will happen.
- Deference to expertise: HROs shift decisions away from formal authority toward expertise and experience. Decision-making migrates to experts at all levels of the hierarchy during high tempo times.

HIGH RELIABILITY ORGANIZATION CHARACTERISTICS*

PREOCCUPATION WITH FAILURE

What is preoccupation with failure?

Preoccupation with failure is a determined mindset to continually watch the system for subtle signs or weak signals of failure. An analogy is the prevention of forest fires: Look for and put out the spark before the fire. Systems with high reliability worry persistently that small errors are rooted in routine work and that unexpected events and limitations of foresight may intensify these errors.

Why is preoccupation with failure important to high reliability?

High reliability means that the expected outcome occurs every time. For example, the outcome of a pilot landing a passenger airplane safely is expected every time. Due to unexpected events and hidden failures, a plane landing successfully once does not mean that it will land successfully in the future. Adverse events in the hospital follow the same course. Adverse events occur in routine and previously successful procedures and processes due to events that were not anticipated and a buildup of hidden or weak failures.

Although success is desirable, it can breed overconfidence and cause blind spots. HROs do not ignore successful operations as resistant to failure. HROs take successful operations and continue to look for and correct unanticipated failures before they occur.

Why is preoccupation with failure challenging to healthcare organizations?

Hospitals need for consumers, staff, and payers to see high-quality care to remain financially viable. Bad news or signs of failure can be perceived as a sign of incompetence or lack of quality. However, adverse events to patients can be prevented when organizations consider "bad news" such as early identification of signs of failure as "good news" because it leads to correction of the problem prior to a total breakdown.

What are some hospital examples of preoccupation with failure?

- Calling the RRT for a subtle sign of clinical deterioration and moving the patient to the ICU prior to a resuscitation
- Reporting near misses and digging deeper to find out why they occur and how the problem could be corrected prior to reaching a patient
- Conducting Failure Mode Effects Analysis (FMEA) prior to and after implementation of new equipment or processes to determine latent or weak failures in the system

Is your unit/work area preoccupied with failure? Ask:

- Are we rewarded when we report mistakes, near misses? Is it easy to report a near miss?
- What near misses were reported here, and did we change anything because of the near miss? Why or why not?

* Weick, K, & Sutcliffe, K. (2015). *Managing the unexpected: Sustained performance in a complex world* (3rd ed.). Jossey-Bass.

RELUCTANCE TO SIMPLIFY

What is reluctance to simplify?

Failures seldom occur without early warning signs. Early warning signs of problems are easily missed when the focus is on quick solutions based on a narrow or predetermined viewpoint. More often, the solution is found within the full context or the details of a situation. *Reluctance to simplify* means that problems are solved by asking more questions from diverse viewpoints to paint a richer picture of the problem. Solutions are generated by refusing to categorize the problem until it is fully described.

Why is reluctance to simplify important to high reliability?

HROs work to become experts at handling unexpected events. Unexpected events come from diverse pathways. Diversity is needed to fully explore the range of these unexpected events. For example, if nursing were the only discipline consulted about a patient care problem, the range of possible solutions would be limited to nursing viewpoints and interventions. This would be simplifying the problem by categorizing it to nursing and ignoring the diversity needed from other disciplines. Problems seldom arise from just one cause, so it is ineffective to try to solve problems with just one discipline or viewpoint.

Why is reluctance to simplify challenging to healthcare organizations?

To simplify means to label or categorize to make a situation actionable. Simplification drives organization life, especially healthcare. Actions in the hospital are based on using metrics and impressions to place a situation into a known category. Reluctance to simplify is difficult, especially in healthcare, because it calls for us to suspend our beliefs and hierarchies to obtain deeper information. That deeper information is often sought in the form of multidisciplinary collaboration in which all disciplines and viewpoints are heard. True multidisciplinary collaboration remains a healthcare challenge.

What are some hospital examples of reluctance to simplify?

- A multidisciplinary group convened to address a system problem.
- Root Cause Analysis that looks at all aspects of a system problem.
- Using data as a jumping-off point to examine issues further. Example: using focus groups to dig deeper into low scores on a Patient Safety Survey.
- Multidisciplinary patient care rounds with emphasis on all disciplines' participation and involvement in problem-solving.

Does your work unit exhibit a reluctance to simplify? Ask:

- Is staff rewarded for asking questions, questioning the status quo, and questioning authority?
- Are people encouraged to bring up difficult problems that have the potential to stop a process or procedure?

SENSITIVITY TO OPERATIONS

What is sensitivity to operations?

Sensitivity to operations means that the organization responds and detects flaws in the system as it exists. In other words, the organization is "responsive to the messy reality" inside the system. Organizations striving for high reliability examine current processes and how real-time staff behaviors are shaped by these processes. For example, when a protocol deviation is noted, the HRO seeks to find out why the protocol was not followed rather than force a protocol that does not rationally work within the context.

Why is sensitivity to operations important to high reliability?

Sensitivity to operations concerns attention paid to how the work *is* done in real time rather than how it *should* be done. Policies, procedures, and protocols can work wonderfully on paper, but the success of these interventions is in the implementation at the work site. For example, workarounds are a symptom of an ineffective process. As workarounds persist, they become normalized, causing the system or process to become more vulnerable to failure. Sensitivity to operations detects workarounds as a symptom of impending failure to prevent this vulnerability.

Why is sensitivity to operations challenging to healthcare organizations?

Analysis of past events is the norm in the healthcare organization. Events are analyzed in terms of what should have been done dependent on existing rules or protocols. This analysis is an example of hindsight bias. Hindsight bias occurs when we already know the outcome and fall back on blaming the problem on user error or "this person did not follow the protocol." Hindsight bias is not helpful because it does not consider the context and why the person did a certain action. Digging deeper into the "why" is often difficult, but digging deeper unearths system causes of error that direct staff nearer to the error. Correcting these system causes is not as easy as correcting the individual, but it will lead to longer-lasting error prevention.

What are some hospital examples of sensitivity to operations?

- Examining why medications were not scanned as defined per protocol
- Examining why a rapid response team was not called when the patient met the criteria

Is your work area sensitive to operations? Ask:

- Do people doing different jobs come into enough contact with each other during the day to have a big picture of how processes are working?
- Do supervisors constantly monitor workload and throughput to ensure that resources are available for busy times or emergencies?

COMMITMENT TO RESILIENCE

What is commitment to resilience?

The Merriam Webster dictionary defines *resilience* as "the ability to recover from or adjust easily to misfortune or change." The current climate of healthcare and patient care is one of change and unexpected events. Organizations that commit to resilience create an environment with resources to quickly shift gears when a change occurs so they can problem-solve, learn, and disseminate the learning and prevent further failure.

Characteristics include:

- Plan for redistributing staff for emergencies
- Ability to improvise and be creative
- Ability to form ad-hoc teams of experts

Why is commitment to resilience important to high reliability?

HROs realize that change and failures are sometimes inevitable. However, catastrophic failure can occur if organizations are not able to shift gears to constrain the damage.

Why is commitment to resilience challenging to healthcare organizations?

A main tenet of resilience is to have resources ready for surprises. Generally, organizations such as hospitals have a historic and financial mindset of preparation for the known rather than the unknown. Preparing for the unknown requires training and preparation for emergencies and a healthy appreciation that bad things do and will happen in situations that have previously been routine.

What are some hospital examples of commitment to resilience?

- Command Center used as a vehicle for hospital collaboration for emergent events
- Immediate healthcare team collaboration or conference for changes in patient condition
- Rapid response team activation for changes in patient condition
- Debriefing of staff after unusual or rare patient care events
- Mock code blue training

Is your work area committed to resilience? Ask:

- What was the last unexpected event that occurred here? Did we have the immediate resources to problem-solve and do what was needed for the patient? Why or why not?
- What did we learn from that event? Is the learning still in practice here?

DEFERENCE TO EXPERTISE

What is deference to expertise?

Deference to expertise means that the organization allows decisions to come from people or teams from all corners of the system. Those closest to the problem are empowered to speak up and call attention to the problem and are empowered to make decisions that affect their work.

Why is deference to expertise important to high reliability?

Deference to authority, as is common in most healthcare operations, is the norm for low-risk, routine operations. However, unexpected situations often arise that the person in authority may not be in a position to recognize. Weak signals of failure are often noted by lower ranking members of the team, thus shifting the level of needed authority to those who are closest to the problem. High reliability depends on those closest to the problem to have the authority and support to speak up, make decisions, and stop a process to preserve patient safety.

Why is deference to expertise challenging to healthcare organizations?

Healthcare organizations typically and historically function in a top-down, hierarchical model, with those at the highest levels easily heard and those at the lowest levels silent. There is also a natural fear of appearing personally incompetent when acknowledging failure. Fear of reporting and structural and cultural hierarchy are two top challenges to deference to expertise.

What are some hospital examples of deference to expertise?

- Multidisciplinary timeouts prior to procedures with the ability for anyone to ask questions in a supportive environment before the start
- Multidisciplinary rounds with input from all providers and support for questions asked
- Executive rounding on nursing units for feedback
- Protocols that allow discretion and summoning of resources at the point of care: Stroke protocol, RRT protocol

Does your work area defer to expertise? Ask:

- Do staff who do the work ask to be involved in decisions that affect their work?
- Do staff in this area value expertise over hierarchical rank or authority?
- Is there respect for the nature of the different jobs that people do here?

www.ingramcontent.com/pod-product-compliance
Lightning Source LLC
Chambersburg PA
CBHW082148300426

44117CB00016B/2660